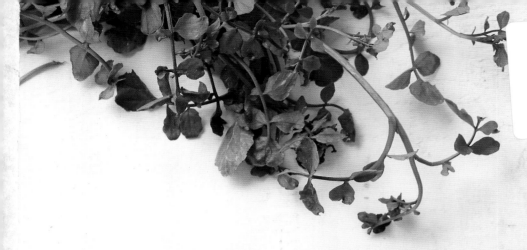

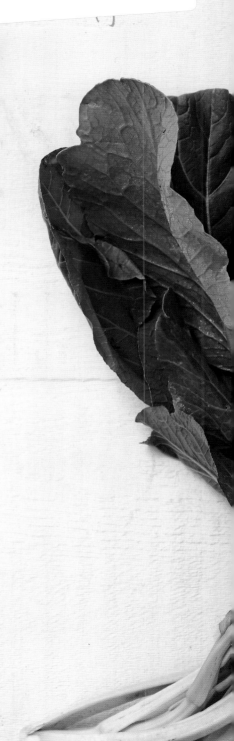

The BUSY MUM'S *guide to* WEIGHT LOSS

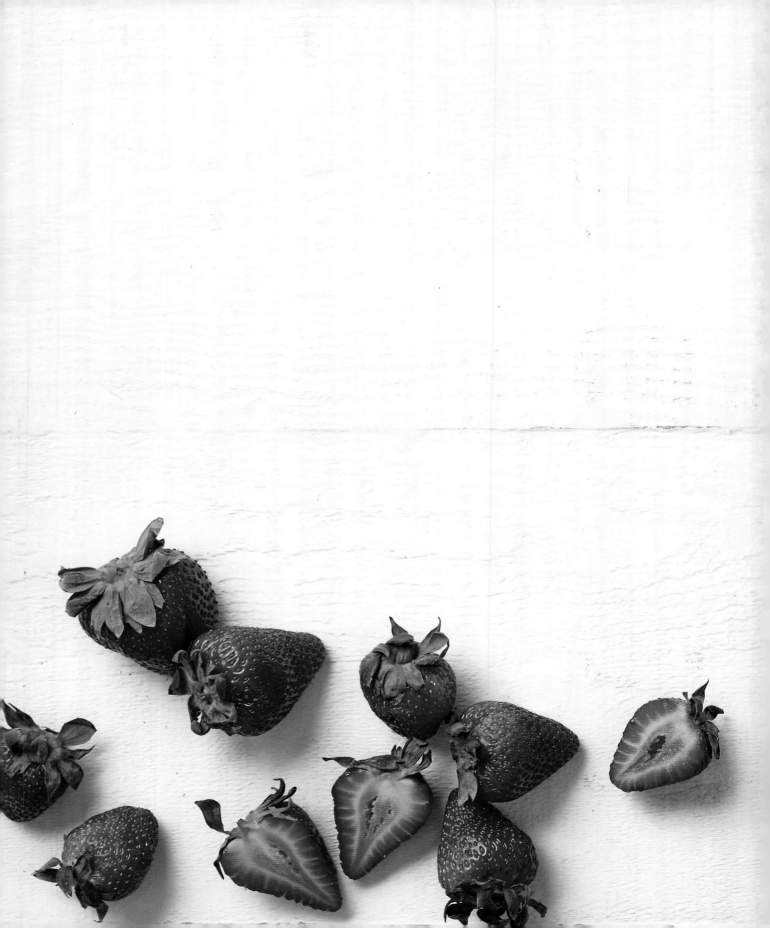

The *BUSY MUM'S* guide to *WEIGHT LOSS*

Rhian Allen

 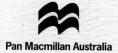

plum. Pan Macmillan Australia

CONTENTS

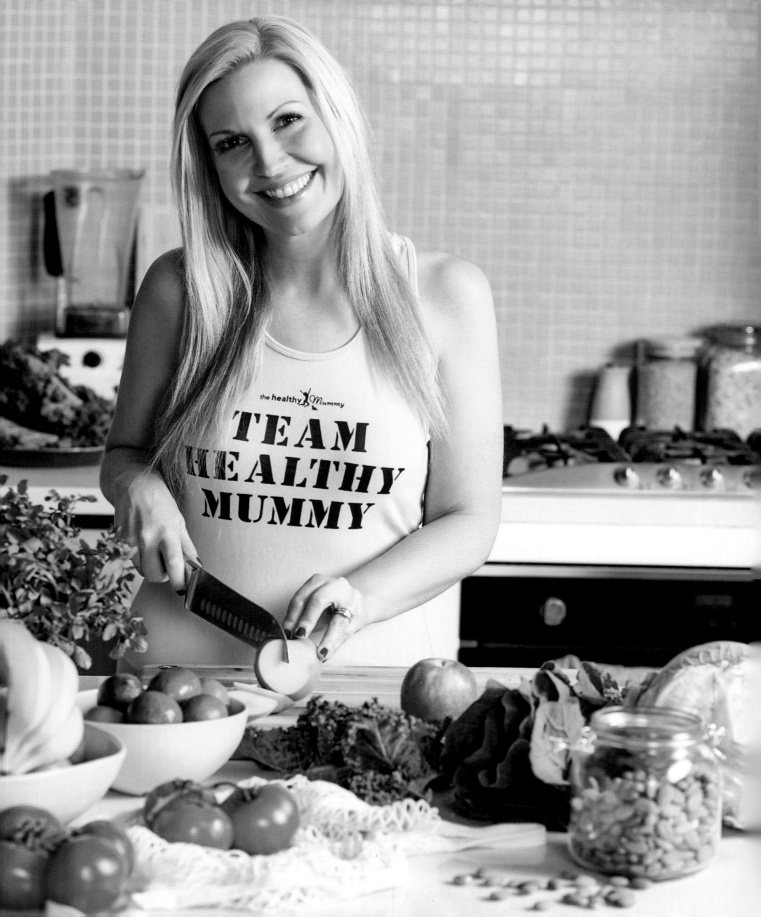

ABOUT THE HEALTHY MUMMY

You may have seen my page pop up on Facebook or heard your friends talk about how they lost weight and regained their body confidence using my 28 Day Weight Loss Challenge app and some of my other products, such as my range of smoothies. But what exactly is The Healthy Mummy?

A few years ago, I started looking for ways to create a holistic and national support system to help mums lose weight and get healthy after giving birth. In 2010 I created The Healthy Mummy website (healthymummy.com) with a simple and achievable 28 day eating and exercise program to help get mums in shape. Since then, The Healthy Mummy has become the biggest mums-only healthy-eating and weight-loss program in Australia – and it's growing EVERY DAY!

The Healthy Mummy weight-loss program aims to empower women to live a healthier life through exercise and family-friendly healthy-eating meal plans on a budget.

But the aim is not for these women to achieve unrealistic weight loss in a short space of time; it's all about encouraging mums to learn about healthy living and healthy food, and doing so in a supportive, inclusive environment.

As a mum of two, I understand that motherhood is demanding and HARD WORK, which is why the recipes, exercises, products and everything involved is tailored to suit a busy mum and a family-friendly environment.

The Busy Mum's Guide to Weight Loss features my favourite recipes and exercises from The Healthy Mummy 28 Day Weight Loss Challenge app, making it even easier to lose weight in a healthy and sustainable way, while still being able to eat delicious meals you and your family will love.

Rhian

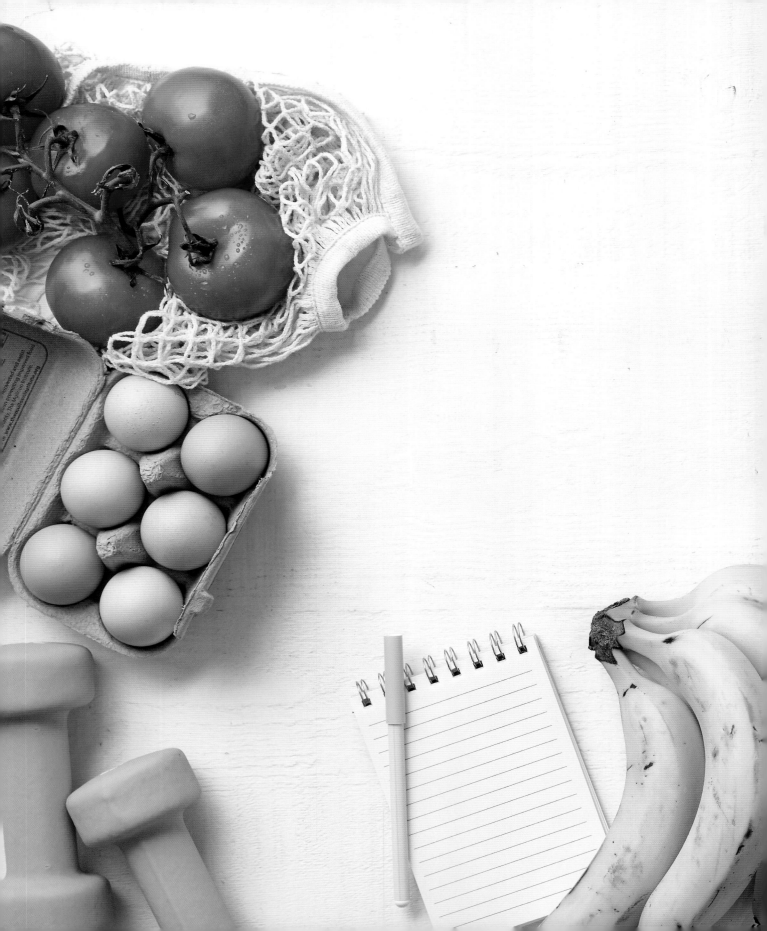

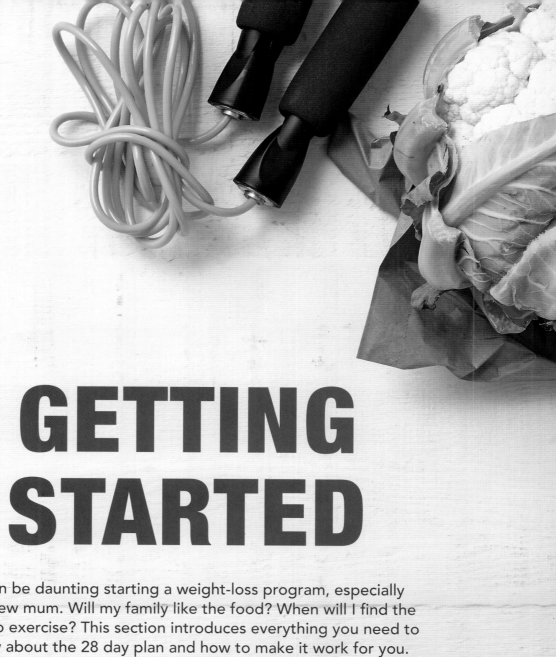

GETTING STARTED

It can be daunting starting a weight-loss program, especially as a new mum. Will my family like the food? When will I find the time to exercise? This section introduces everything you need to know about the 28 day plan and how to make it work for you.

WHAT IS THE 28 DAY PLAN?

Developed by The Healthy Mummy's team of nutritionists and fitness experts, the 28 day plan has been designed specifically for busy, budget-conscious mums to help them lose weight in a healthy way and take charge of their health. It consists of two elements, the 28 day meal plan and the 28 day exercise plan.

The 28 day meal plan aims to help mums prepare healthy, affordable and timesaving dishes that the whole family can enjoy. What's more, the meals within the plans can be swapped out to suit personal tastes and dietary preferences.

The 28 day exercise plan contains daily exercises, along with suggestions developed by our postnatal exercise expert to help mums lose weight and tone up safely. These workouts do not require equipment and can therefore be performed in the comfort of your own home (and with a baby on the hip).

The 28 day plan is NOT about deprivation. It's about eating a healthy balanced diet and moving more. It's about implementing healthy lifestyle changes that stick.

On the 28 day plan you can expect to lose between 500 g and 1 kg a week. You can even follow the plan if you are breastfeeding. In fact, many of the foods on the plan have been specifically selected to support breast-milk supply.

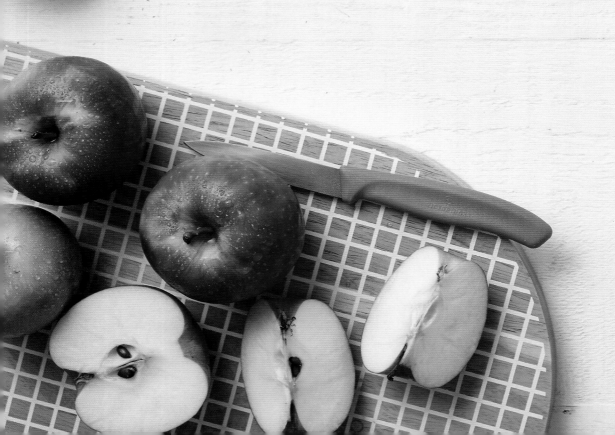

HOW THE MEAL PLAN WORKS

The Healthy Mummy weekly meal plan isn't restrictive and allows you to consume approximately 1400–1500 calories per day.

But depending on your personal basal metabolic rate (BMR), you may need to increase or decrease portion sizes accordingly. You could also try adding extra snacks to ensure that you are eating to suit your personal energy requirements (see 'Getting Started – BMR' on page 13 for further details).

The meal plan is full of variety to suit individual tastes and you don't need to follow it rigidly; use it as a guide to suit your needs. For instance, if you follow a gluten- or dairy-free diet you can easily swap ingredients. You might also like to make extra serves and store them in the fridge or freezer for another meal.

Some people prefer to repeat meals during the week. For example, choose a couple of breakfast recipes to have throughout the week rather than something different every day, or plan to have leftovers from dinner for lunch the next day. This will help you save time and money.

And if you don't like a certain food, such as seafood, just replace it with a lean protein you do like. However, we do encourage you to try some new flavours while following the plan to ensure that your diet is well balanced and you are eating a wide variety of nutrients.

Snack recipes are usually made in larger batches to eat throughout the week. We've also included a selection of smoothie recipes that can be used as meal replacements (for example, for breakfast or as a snack).

Each recipe includes a comprehensive nutritional breakdown per serve, which includes calories, kilojoules, protein, fibre, total fat, saturated fat, carbohydrates, total sugar and free sugar (added sugar).

The meal plan includes a variety of key nutrients for a healthy body, including the following:

PROTEIN

Protein is vital for the growth, maintenance and repair of cells. Protein-rich foods, such as meat, chicken, fish, legumes, tofu, nuts and dairy, help you feel satisfied by keeping hunger at bay for longer. Aim to include protein-rich foods in every meal and snack.

CALCIUM

Dairy foods, such as milk, cheese and yoghurt provide the richest sources of calcium. Other good sources include fish (for example, salmon and sardines), tofu, seeds and nuts. Many women do not meet the recommended daily intake for calcium. Aim for 3 serves of calcium-rich foods a day, although breastfeeding women may require up to 4 serves a day to protect bone strength. We advise you to choose low-fat varieties where possible, as they will be lower in calories.

CARBOHYDRATES

Include low glycemic index (GI) carbohydrates at each meal and snack, to keep your energy levels up and blood sugar levels stable.

DIETARY FIBRE

Eating a high-fibre diet helps maintain digestive health and will keep you feeling full on fewer calories.

THE PLAN AND BREASTFEEDING

Your body burns up a lot of energy (calories/kilojoules) to make breast milk, particularly for mothers who are exclusively breastfeeding.

On average, nursing mums following the 28 day plan should add an extra 500 calories (2200 kJ) per day on top of their usual energy needs. You can do this by having a couple of additional healthy snacks, a smoothie or a larger portion for main meals.

If you are trying to lose weight while breastfeeding, it's important to aim for a gradual weight loss of around 500 g per week. A steady weight loss back to pre-pregnancy weight should be the goal, rather than rapid weight loss, keeping the focus on eating a healthy, balanced diet.

Certain nutrients, energy and fluids will be in high demand while you are breastfeeding, much more than during pregnancy. These include the following:

IRON

Iron is a mineral that contains a number of proteins, including haemoglobin, which is important for transporting oxygen around the body. Red meat, chicken and fish are great sources of iron, as well as being good sources of protein and zinc. Iron can also be found in green leafy vegetables and legumes. To increase the amount of iron the body absorbs, it should be consumed with foods rich in vitamin C (such as tomato, broccoli or capsicum). If you eat too little iron, you will suffer from fatigue and have a weakened immune system.

IODINE

Because breast milk needs to contain adequate iodine levels to support your infant's growing brain, a new mother's iodine requirements are almost double the normal level. Good sources of iodine include bread, iodised salt, seafood, eggs and dairy but, in addition, supplements containing iodine are usually recommended. Make sure you speak to your doctor before taking any supplements.

ZINC

Zinc is essential for immune function, skin health and optimal reproductive health. Good sources of zinc include meat, breakfast cereals, brightly coloured vegetables and fruit.

WATER

Water is the best way to quench your thirst and it doesn't contain the added sugar and calories found in sweetened drinks, such as fruit juices, soft drinks, sports drinks and flavoured mineral waters. While water doesn't increase milk production, it is still important to keep hydrated. A good guide is to drink a glass at each meal and again with each breastfeed.

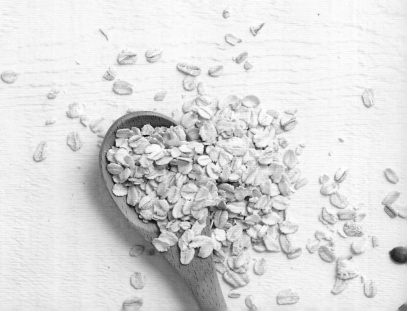

GETTING STARTED

BMR

Your basal metabolic rate (BMR) is the number of calories you'd burn if you sat there all day and didn't do a thing. It's a really important number to know, for a couple of reasons.

Firstly, your BMR indicates how much you can eat and still lose weight. Secondly, it gives you an idea of how much you must eat to stay healthy.

Eating significantly less than your BMR calories is NOT recommended as this can send your body into energy-conserving starvation mode (meaning no fat loss).

Your BMR decreases as you age, which is why many of us find it harder to lose weight as we get older. However, the good news is that you can increase your BMR with a regular routine of cardiovascular exercise, muscle-building exercises and metabolism-boosting foods.

As a guide to minimum calorie intake, we would recommend your base level never drops below 1200 calories per day for women or 1800 calories per day for men. It is also important that the calories you consume are nutrient-dense. This will help provide your body with essential vitamins and minerals.

Men and women have to use different equations to determine their BMR. This is based on the assumption that men have a higher percentage of lean body weight than women (more lean body weight = increased BMR).

Use the formula below to work out your BMR calorie requirements:

Women

BMR = 655 + (9.6 x your weight in kg) + (1.9 x your height in cm) – (4.7 x your age in years)

Men

BMR = 67 + (13.75 x your weight in kg) + (5 x your height in cm) – (6.8 x your age in years)

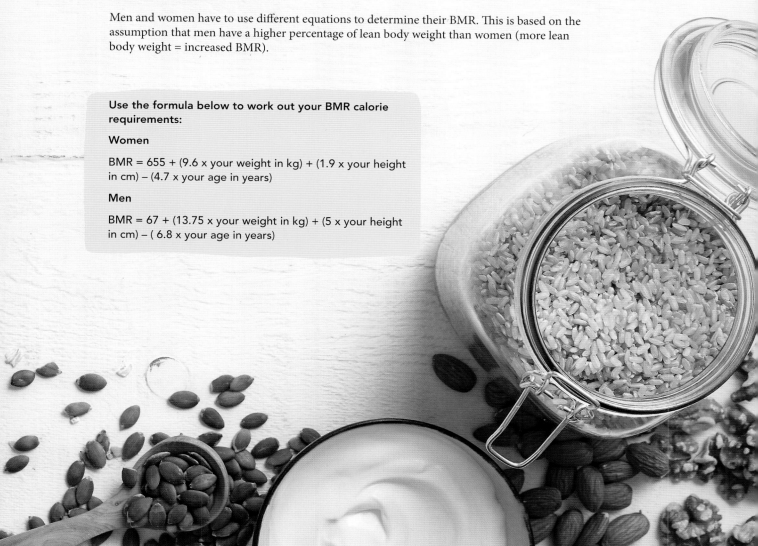

There is also a formula for working out your daily energy calorie needs. These are the calories your body needs AFTER taking into account your BMR and how much exercise you currently do.

To work out what your total daily calorie needs are, you need to multiply your BMR by the activity factor below that suits your current lifestyle:

If you are sedentary (little or no exercise), multiply your BMR by 1.1.

If you are lightly active (light exercise/sports 1–3 days per week), multiply your BMR by 1.275.

If you are moderately active (moderate exercise/sports 3–5 days per week), multiply your BMR by 1.35.

If you are very active (hard exercise/sports 6–7 days per week), multiply your BMR by 1.525.

The figure you now have is the total number of daily calories you need to maintain your current weight. Before starting the 28 day plan, reduce this figure by 10–15 per cent to calculate how many calories you should aim to consume each day to lose weight.

Bear in mind this is just a guide, and results may vary between individuals. If you are hungry while following the plan then eat more, but if you're completely full, eat less (for example, by eliminating one of the daily snacks).

BMI

Body mass index (BMI) is a measurement that uses a scientific formula to determine a person's safest, healthiest weight based upon their weight and height. Having a high BMI can be associated with serious health risks including obesity, heart disease, diabetes and cancer.

Use the formula below to work out your BMI:

Calculate your weight in kilograms (for example, 65 kg)

Take your height in metres (for example, 1.6 m) and square it – so 1.6 m x 1.6 m = 2.56

Then divide your weight by your height squared – so 65 ÷ 2.56 = 23

Your BMI is 23

WHAT DO THE RESULTS OF THE BMI CALCULATOR MEAN?

You can interpret your BMI results as follows:

Below 20: slender, lean (possibly no need to follow this plan as you have probably reached your weight-loss goal).

20 to 25: ideal weight range (you might want to follow this plan to reach your final weight-loss goal or break through a weight-loss plateau).

25 to 30: overweight; 25–27 could be a healthy range for those who are large-boned and heavily muscled (this plan could help you to break through a weight-loss plateau or lose the final few kilos to get you into your ideal weight range).

30 and above: very overweight/high risk for health complications (this plan should only be followed after speaking to your medical professionals to determine if it is right for you).

40 and above: extremely overweight/high risk for health complications (this plan should only be followed after speaking to your medical professionals to determine if it is right for you).

Please note that BMI results should be used as a guide only.

SET YOUR GOALS

There's more to losing weight (and keeping it off) than the food you're putting in your mouth or the amount of exercise you do. The mental component behind weight loss is JUST as important. If you're not in the right headspace to focus on weight loss, the chances are that it just won't happen.

This book is here to help you get into the right frame of mind to achieve your wellness goals. A good way to start is to really think about what you want from the 28 day plan, then set specific goals to keep you focused.

We recommend sticking to the SMART system:

SPECIFIC: 'I want to lose 4 kg' instead of 'I want to lose weight'.
MEASURABLE: 'I will go to bed at 9 pm each night' rather than 'I will go to bed earlier'.
ATTAINABLE: 'I will walk 30 minutes a day, 3 days a week' instead of 'I will exercise 4 hours every day'.
RELEVANT: 'I want to fit into my wedding dress' rather than 'I won't eat Nutella from the jar any more'.
TIME-BOUND: 'I want to lose 3–4 kg a month' instead of 'I want to lose weight fast'.

Below are some other great SMART goals that you might hope to achieve.

In the next 28 days:

- I am going to lose 2 cm from my arms
- I am going to swap white rice for brown rice
- I am going to swap all soft drinks for water
- I am going to dedicate 20 minutes a week to swimming
- I am going to make sure I am in bed by 10 pm every night
- I am going to set aside 15 minutes every 3–4 days to write in my calendar and organise my meals
- I am going to swap milk chocolate for dark chocolate (no less than 70 per cent cocoa solids)

PLAN YOUR REWARDS

Once you've set your goals, set some rewards! We don't recommend rewarding yourself with food, but here are some other ideas:

- Go to the movies
- Organise a date night with your partner
- Book a girls' weekend away
- Buy yourself new active wear
- Head to the hairdresser and reward yourself with a new look
- Shout yourself a new outfit

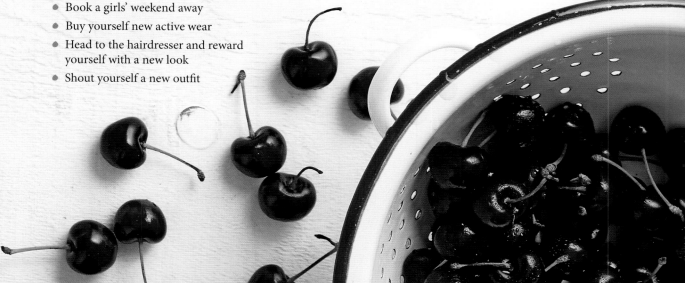

TIMESAVING AND PLANNING

When it comes to getting organised, the 28 day meal plan has done a lot of the hard work for you. The plan includes everything you need to complete the weekly recipes, including shopping lists, so you will no longer come home and panic about an empty fridge and not have a clue what to cook for dinner.

To totally bullet-proof your 28 day meal plan, follow these helpful tips.

CALENDAR PLANNING

Get yourself a calendar – a big family planner for the fridge or use the calendar on your mobile, whatever works for you – and write in all the activities you need to be aware of each week. For example, when are the kids at daycare? Dentist appointments? Working days? Any upcoming social events? This will help clarify what meals need to be organised and when.

SCHEDULE IN PLANNING TIME

Give yourself 15 minutes every 3–4 days to do your planning. Pop this in your calendar if you need to. Write down an idea of what you have available to eat, when you are going to head to the shops and what you will need to prepare each week.

GO THROUGH THE WEEKLY MEAL PLAN AND SHOPPING LIST

Start with what you already have – it helps if you can manage to keep an orderly pantry and a well-stocked fridge and freezer with food in clearly labelled stackable containers. Do you have any frozen healthy meals that you can just thaw and reheat? Do you already have most of the ingredients for certain recipes so you don't need to buy as much? Do you have lots of leftover fruit or vegetables or other ingredients from the previous week that you could use as swaps in other recipes to save time and money?

DOUBLE UP TO SAVE TIME

To make your life easier, consider which meals you can make that will save you time later, whether it's for next week or lunch the next day. Buy double the ingredients so you can cook up a storm! Recipes that are great for freezing include soups, pasta sauces and bakes, stews, curries, burger patties, rice dishes and healthy sweet snacks, such as bliss balls and slices.

PRE-PREPARE TO SAVE TIME

A freezer full of meals is a lifesaver on super-busy nights, but you can also make your life easier by doing a bit of *mise en place* at home, prepping your ingredients as you put them away. You might want to chop veggies for stir-fries or snacks and wash salad leaves; trim and marinate meats before putting them in freezer bags; or cook brown rice or quinoa and freeze in individual portions, to be thawed and reheated as required.

RECRUIT THE FAMILY

If you can get your family involved with food preparation, it will save you loads of time and also make them more interested in the food they are eating. Depending on their ages, kids can do a lot of things in the kitchen to help out: chopping vegetables and fruit, stirring pots, measuring and adding ingredients. Many hands make light work, so if everyone does a few tasks, the cooking will be done in next to no time.

TIPS FOR STAYING ON BUDGET

It's not unusual for mums to worry about the cost of healthy eating, with many thinking it is an expensive way to go. That may be true for pre-made meals and snacks, but you can be smart about what you buy on a budget!

Here are some easy tips to follow while on the 28 day meal plan to keep your healthy lifestyle on budget:

MENU PLAN

The menu planning has already been done for you on the 28 day meal plan and you can customise it to suit your family, budget and tastes. You don't have to choose a different meal for each day of the week either; you can repeat some of your breakfast options, make extra dinners to have for lunch the next day or choose just a couple of easy-to-prepare snacks, which will not only save you money but also reduce your meal-prep times.

BUY IN BULK

Products such as meats, frozen foods, flours, rice, grains and other pantry staples are great to buy in bulk, saving you a substantial amount of money in the long term. Wholesalers often sell staples, such as pasta, rice, tinned goods and condiments that are great value for money.

BUY FROZEN

Frozen fruits and vegetables are cheap and often on special. They're also good quality as they are usually picked and frozen within 24 hours.

BE SMART WITH YOUR SHOPPING

You can also customise the shopping lists (see page 18). Take stock of what you have in the pantry, fridge and freezer and use the ingredients already available to you. Swap ingredients so they don't go to waste or use up the vegetables you already have rather than buy specific ones to use in a recipe. Use the shopping list guides in the meal plans to write your shopping list, then take it to the shops and only purchase what's on that list!

USE YOUR FREEZER

Where possible, use your freezer to store food you've purchased in bulk. Vegetables, such as corn on the cob, sliced carrots, peas, green beans, broccoli and cauliflower last much longer this way. You can either buy these from the frozen section or freeze your own in ziplock bags. Double your recipes and freeze half for another time. If you don't have a huge freezer, portion meals in ziplock bags so they can be stored flat in the freezer to save space.

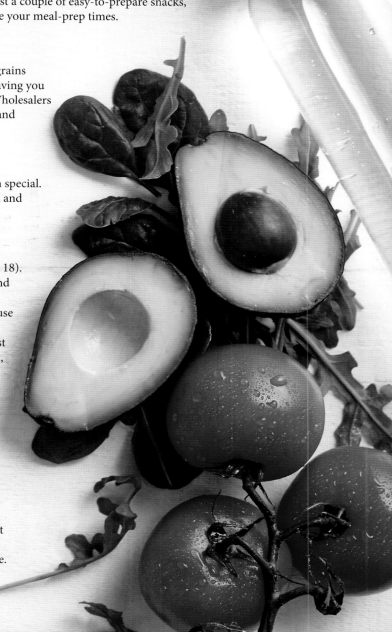

BUY IN SEASON AND BUY LOCAL

As a rule, produce tastes better and is much cheaper when it is in season. Buying local also benefits the environment and local economy. More often than not the quality is far superior too, meaning you won't be throwing away any rotting vegetables at the end of the week.

SHOP AROUND

While major supermarkets are convenient for stocking up on a wide variety of products, they aren't always the cheapest places to do your shopping. Buying fresh produce at your local farmers' market or greengrocer can often save you money. Many local butchers and fishmongers sell in bulk at a discounted rate, so shop around and don't be afraid to ask for a bulk discount – just be sure you have enough room in your freezer!

REDUCE WASTE

Save on waste by trying to buy only what you will use and, where possible, buy non-perishable alternatives, such as frozen food.

DON'T SHOP HUNGRY

Everything seems more tempting and delicious when you are hungry, and you may be tempted to make poor food choices or buy more than you need, so don't do it!

SHOP ONLINE

Try shopping online to stop yourself from loading up your trolley with impulse buys. Most major supermarkets offer free click and collect options, which can be a great way to save time and money. You can also easily compare pricing, something that isn't always possible mid-shop with a screaming toddler.

CHECK PRICE PER UNIT

Be aware that the cheapest item on display may not actually be the one with the lowest final price. Make sure you check the 'price per unit' or 'price per 100 g' when comparing products. Supermarkets are required to list this on the price docket – usually in teeny writing at the bottom – so use it to make an informed choice.

SHOPPING LISTS

The 28 day meal plan has a shopping list of fresh foods required to make the recipes each week. A list of pantry staples is also provided at the start of the program (see pages 22–23), and this covers general items needed for the recipes over the 4 weeks. You may need to top up some of these as you progress through the plan.

Before you commence the plan, we suggest you go through the pantry staples list and see which items you already have, then add any remaining ingredients to your shopping list.

Go through the weekly meal plans before you head to the shops to see if there are any recipes you'd like to alter, increase in quantity, swap ingredients and so on. You can then customise the shopping list to suit your needs.

Remember to do a fridge and pantry stocktake each week before doing the next shop as you may have ingredients left over that you can use up or substitute in recipes. This will help reduce waste and save you money.

CARVING OUT TIME FOR EXERCISE

Exercise is important not only for weight loss, but also for general physical health and for mental wellbeing. However, it tends to be the first thing that falls off a busy schedule.

Here are some great tips to ensure you are able to SQUEEZE IN EXERCISE, no matter how busy you are:

SCHEDULE EXERCISE EVERY DAY

Put your workouts in your calendar like any other appointment. This will help you stick to your plan and let the rest of the family know your time is booked. The 28 day plan has an exercise workout/activity scheduled every day to make it really easy for you to know what to do and set aside enough time to complete each task.

GET UP 30 MINUTES EARLIER

Doing exercise first thing in the morning is great for your metabolism and will help put you in a good mood for the rest of the day. If you leave exercise until the end of the day it's sometimes easier to make excuses or allow your time to be hijacked by other commitments.

HIIT IT!

High-intensity interval training is great for busy mums, as you can do short bursts of really beneficial, calorie-burning exercises. You might want to start the day with 10 minutes of one of the HIIT workouts from the 28 day plan, then do another couple of rounds throughout the day. Even if you only manage one round of 10 minutes, that's awesome!

JUST DO SOMETHING

If you've been unwell or unable to stick to your daily exercise plan, just commit to an easy 20-minute walk around the neighbourhood. You won't need equipment or the car to drive anywhere, and it's a great way to get moving (and motivated).

YOU CAN EXERCISE ANYWHERE

When you're really pushed for time, try to fit in some extra incidental exercise throughout the day. Whether it's doing a few squats while waiting for the kettle to boil or some lunges after hanging out the washing, you'll be surprised at how it all adds up and helps you reach your healthy weight-loss goals.

Now that you've set your goals, worked out your daily energy needs to lose weight and planned your meals, you are ready to get started with Week 1!

The recommended exercises for each day are listed on the 28 day meal plan overview pages located at the start of each week. The workouts themselves can be found towards the back of this book, starting on page 276.

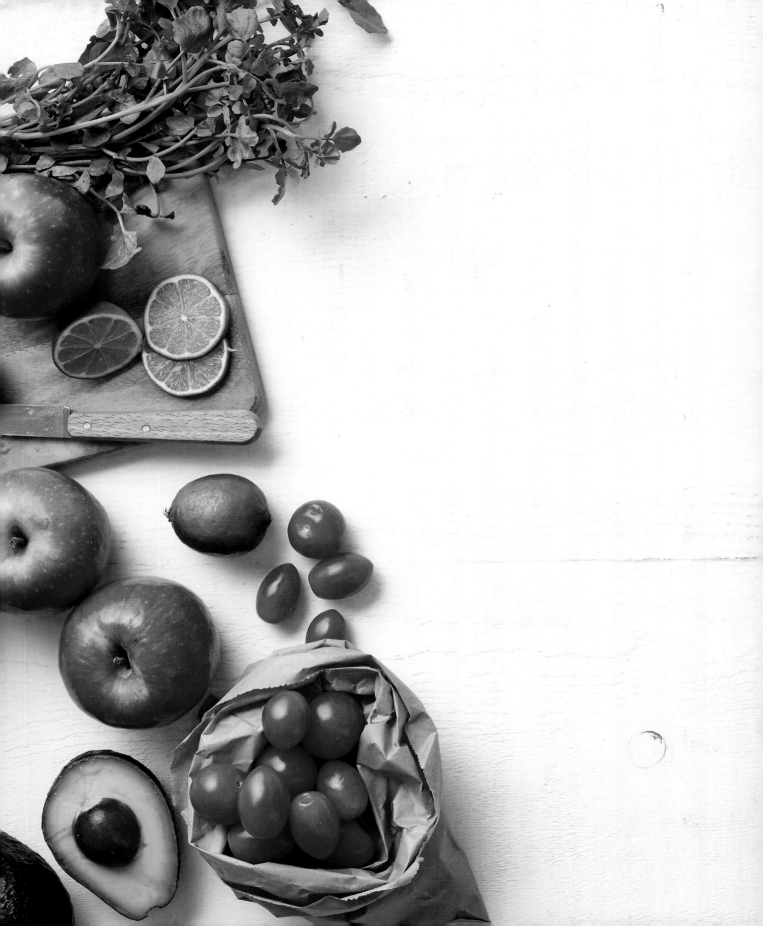

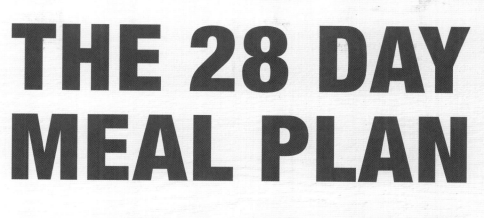

THE 28 DAY MEAL PLAN

Created by The Healthy Mummy's team of nutritional experts, this section contains everything you need to complete the 28 day meal plan with confidence. Refer to the weekly meal and exercise overiew pages to see at a glance what you will be doing each week, and use our handy shopping lists to note down all the ingredients you will need to buy. The pantry list on pages 22–23 contains all the non-perishable goods you will need for the 28 days, while the shopping lists at the start of each week list all the fresh ingredients you need to buy that week.

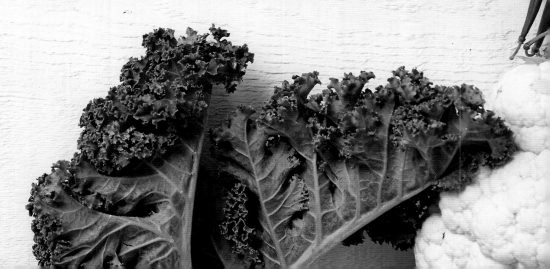

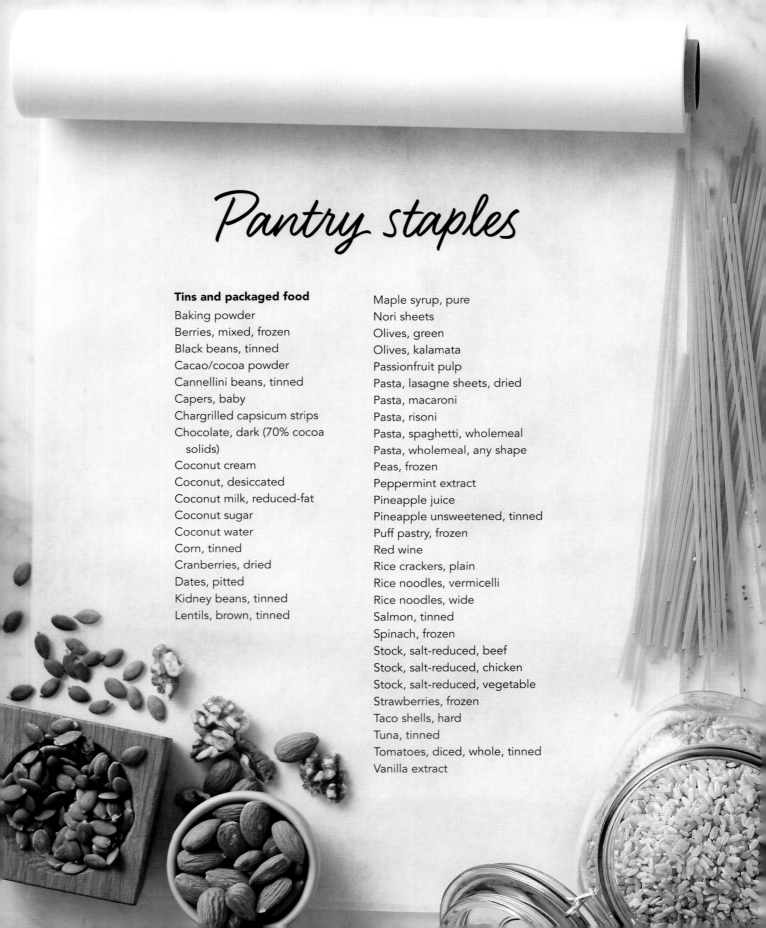

Pantry staples

Tins and packaged food

Baking powder
Berries, mixed, frozen
Black beans, tinned
Cacao/cocoa powder
Cannellini beans, tinned
Capers, baby
Chargrilled capsicum strips
Chocolate, dark (70% cocoa
    solids)
Coconut cream
Coconut, desiccated
Coconut milk, reduced-fat
Coconut sugar
Coconut water
Corn, tinned
Cranberries, dried
Dates, pitted
Kidney beans, tinned
Lentils, brown, tinned

Maple syrup, pure
Nori sheets
Olives, green
Olives, kalamata
Passionfruit pulp
Pasta, lasagne sheets, dried
Pasta, macaroni
Pasta, risoni
Pasta, spaghetti, wholemeal
Pasta, wholemeal, any shape
Peas, frozen
Peppermint extract
Pineapple juice
Pineapple unsweetened, tinned
Puff pastry, frozen
Red wine
Rice crackers, plain
Rice noodles, vermicelli
Rice noodles, wide
Salmon, tinned
Spinach, frozen
Stock, salt-reduced, beef
Stock, salt-reduced, chicken
Stock, salt-reduced, vegetable
Strawberries, frozen
Taco shells, hard
Tuna, tinned
Tomatoes, diced, whole, tinned
Vanilla extract

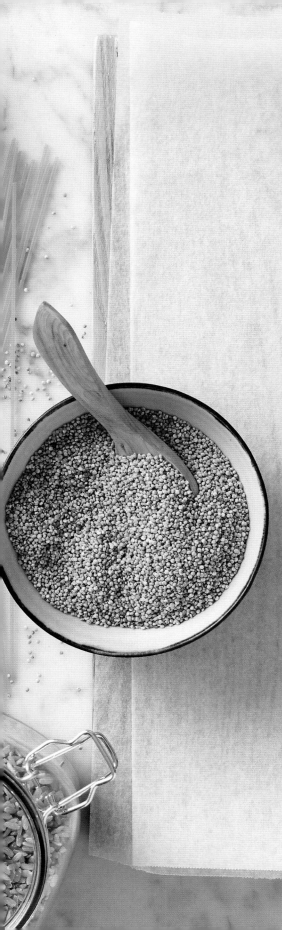

Breads, grains, cereals and nuts

Almond meal
Almonds, whole, natural
Breadcrumbs, dried, wholemeal
Cashews, unsalted
Chia seeds
Cornflour
Couscous
Flour, chickpea (besan)
Flour, plain, wholemeal
Flour, self-raising, wholemeal
Flour, spelt
LSA
Muesli, untoasted
Peanuts
Pistachios, unsalted
Pumpkin seeds
Quinoa
Rice, arborio
Rice, brown
Rice, sushi
Rolled oats
Sesame seeds, black or white
Sunflower seeds
Walnuts

Sauces and pastes

Barbecue sauce, no added sugar
Curry paste, laksa
Curry paste, red
Curry paste, tandoori
Fish sauce
Kecap manis (Indonesian sweet
   soy sauce)
Miso paste
Passata (pureed tomatoes)
Soy sauce
Sweet chilli sauce
Tomato paste
Worcestershire sauce

Dairy

Butter
Greek-style yoghurt, natural,
   reduced-fat
Milk, reduced fat

Spices and condiments

Balsamic vinegar
Basil, dried
Black peppercorns
Chilli flakes
Chilli powder
Cinnamon, ground
Cumin, ground
Cumin seeds
Dill, dried
Honey
Italian herbs, dried
Mayonnaise
Mustard, Dijon
Mustard, wholegrain
Oregano, dried
Paprika, smoked
Peanut butter
Red wine vinegar
Rosemary, dried
Sea salt
Sumac
Taco seasoning, salt-reduced
Tahini
Thyme, dried
Tomato salsa
Turmeric, ground

Oils

Coconut oil
Cooking oil spray
Olive oil, extra virgin
Sesame oil

Tea

Chamomile tea bags
Green tea bags
Matcha green tea powder

WEEK 1.

MEAL & EXERCISE PLAN

1.

	MONDAY	TUESDAY	WEDNESDAY
BREAKFAST	Bacon and Egg Muffins **p.30** 234 cals	Easy Apple and Cinnamon Porridge **p.32** 337 cals	Breakfast Quinoa Salad **p.34** 362 cals
MORNING SNACK	Mexican Layered Dip **p.72** 208 cals	Peanut Butter and Chocolate Cookies **p.74** 147 cals	Lemon and Coconut Bliss Balls **p.76** 171 cals
LUNCH	Chargrilled Capsicum, Olive and Cheese Toasted Sandwich **p.44** 297 cals	Brown Rice and Raw Veg Power Salad **p.46** 353 cals	Detox Soup **p.48** 135 cals
EXERCISE	16 minute Tummy Tamer*, Workout 1 (see page 280)	20 minute Body Strong Pilates, Workout 1 (see page 286)	20 minute Deep Core Conditioning*, Workout 1 (see page 290)
AFTERNOON SNACK	Peanut Butter and Chocolate Cookies **p.74** 147 cals	Lemon and Coconut Bliss Balls **p.76** 171 cals	Mexican Layered Dip **p.72** 208 cals
DINNER	Coconut Lamb with Caulifllower Rice **p.58** 397 cals	Pork with Kiwi Fruit and Watercress Salad **p.61** 418 cals	Chicken Noodle Stir-fry **p.62** 282 cals
EVENING SNACK	Strawberry Cheesecake Ice Blocks **p.80** 149 cals	1 orange served with 1 cup of herbal tea 54 cals	Strawberry Cheesecake Ice Blocks **p.80** 149 cals
TOTAL CALORIES	**1432 cals**	**1480 cals**	**1307 cals**

THURSDAY	FRIDAY	SATURDAY	SUNDAY
Choc–Oat Granola **p.37** 330 cals	BLT Pita Melt **p.38** **277 cals**	Oat and Cinnamon Pancakes **p.40** 289 cals	Salmon Rosti **p.42** 252 cals
Carrot and Avocado Handrolls **p.79** 149 cals	Peanut Butter and Chocolate Cookies **p.74** 147 cals	Mexican Layered Dip **p.72** 208 cals	Peanut Butter and Chocolate Cookies **p.74** 147 cals
Prosciutto, Apple and Rocket Salad **p.50** 205 cals	Corn and Quinoa Fritters **p.51** 348 cals	Easy Pizza Wraps **p.54** 323 cals	Autumn Minestrone **p.57** 333 cals
Low Impact 12 minute Total Body Tabata Workout (see page 294)	20 minute Butt and Thigh*, Workout 1 (see page 298)	20 minute Fat Blaster, Workout 1 (see page 302)	Active Recovery Day 1 (see page 304)
Lemon and Coconut Bliss Balls **p.76** 171 cals	Mexican Layered Dip **p.72** 208 cals	Carrot and Avocado Handrolls **p.79** 149 cals	Carrot and Avocado Handrolls **p.79** 149 cals
Mexican Lasagne **p.64** 483 cals	Fish and Veggie Kebabs **p.66** 286 cals	Zoodles with Haloumi and Roasted Vegetables **p.69** 272 cals	Loaded Sweet Potato Fries **p.70** 397 cals
Peanut Butter and Chocolate Cookies **p.74** 147 cals	Lemon and Coconut Bliss Balls **p.76** 171 cals	Lemon and Coconut Bliss Balls **p.76** 171 cals	Strawberry Cheesecake Ice Blocks **p.80** 149 cals
1485 cals	**1437 cals**	**1412 cals**	**1427 cals**

*Choose the low-impact variation of this workout if you are still recovering from a C-section, abdominal separation, prolapse, or if you have a weak pelvic floor.

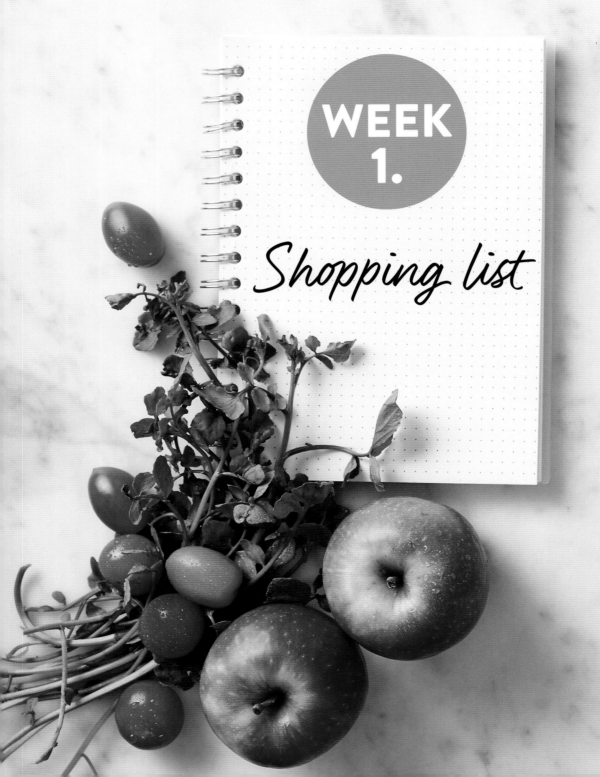

WEEK 1.

Shopping list

Vegetables

Baby spinach leaves 50 g
Bok choy (2) 300 g
Broccoli 600 g
Capsicums, red 8
Carrots 8
Cauliflower 1 kg
Celery ½ bunch
Corn kernels 100 g (or use tinned)
Garlic 15 cloves
Ginger 1 small knob
Kale 120 g
Lettuce leaves, mixed 2 cups
Mushrooms, small 450 g
Mushrooms, large flat 200 g
Onions, brown 3
Onions, red 3
Potatoes 2
Rocket leaves 120 g
Spring onions 6
Sweet potatoes 4 small
Tomatoes 6
Tomatoes, roma 4
Watercress 80 g
Zucchini 12

Fruit

Apples, red 3
Avocados 4
Banana 1
Blueberries 150 g
Kiwi fruit 2
Lemons 6
Limes 3
Oranges 3

Fresh herbs

Coriander 1 bunch
Dill 1 sprig
Flat-leaf parsley 2 bunches
Mint 1 sprig
Rosemary 1 sprig
Thyme 2 sprigs

Meat, fish and poultry

Bacon rashers, lean and
    trimmed (8) 200 g
Beef mince, lean 400 g
Chicken breast fillets 400 g
Eggs, free-range 10
Fish fillets, white 600 g
Ham, lean smoked 120 g
Lamb steak, lean 400 g
Pork fillet 400 g
Prosciutto, sliced 120 g

Dairy

Cheddar, reduced-fat 250 g
Cream cheese, light 130 g
Feta, reduced-fat 30 g
Haloumi 160 g
Parmesan, shaved 80 g
Ricotta, reduced-fat 170 g
Yoghurt, reduced-fat natural
    Greek-style 180 g

Breads and grains

Bread of choice, wholemeal
    or gluten free, 6 slices
Mountain bread wraps,
    wholemeal 4
Pita bread, wholemeal 2
Tortillas, wholemeal 5

BACON AND EGG MUFFINS

SERVES: 2   **PREPARATION TIME:** 10 MINUTES   **COOKING TIME:** 20–25 MINUTES

cooking oil spray
4 free-range eggs
2 tablespoons reduced-fat milk
of choice
4 lean bacon rashers, trimmed
¼ red onion, chopped
¼ red capsicum, seeds
removed, chopped
1 tablespoon grated
reduced-fat cheddar
flat-leaf parsley leaves,
to garnish

Preheat the oven to 180°C. Lightly spray four holes of a standard muffin tin with cooking oil spray and line with baking paper or patty pan cases.

Beat the eggs and milk and set aside.

Line each of the prepared muffin holes with a spiralled rasher of bacon. Divide the onion and capsicum among the holes, then evenly pour in the egg mixture and sprinkle over the grated cheese.

Bake for 20–25 minutes or until the egg is set. Divide between two plates and serve hot, sprinkled with the parsley and freshly ground pepper, if desired.

NUTRI DETAILS PER SERVE

234 cals/983 kjs
Protein: 23.4 g
Fibre: 0.3 g
Total fat: 14.3 g
Sat fat: 4.6 g
Carbs: 3.3 g
Total sugar: 2.7 g
Free sugar: 0.0 g

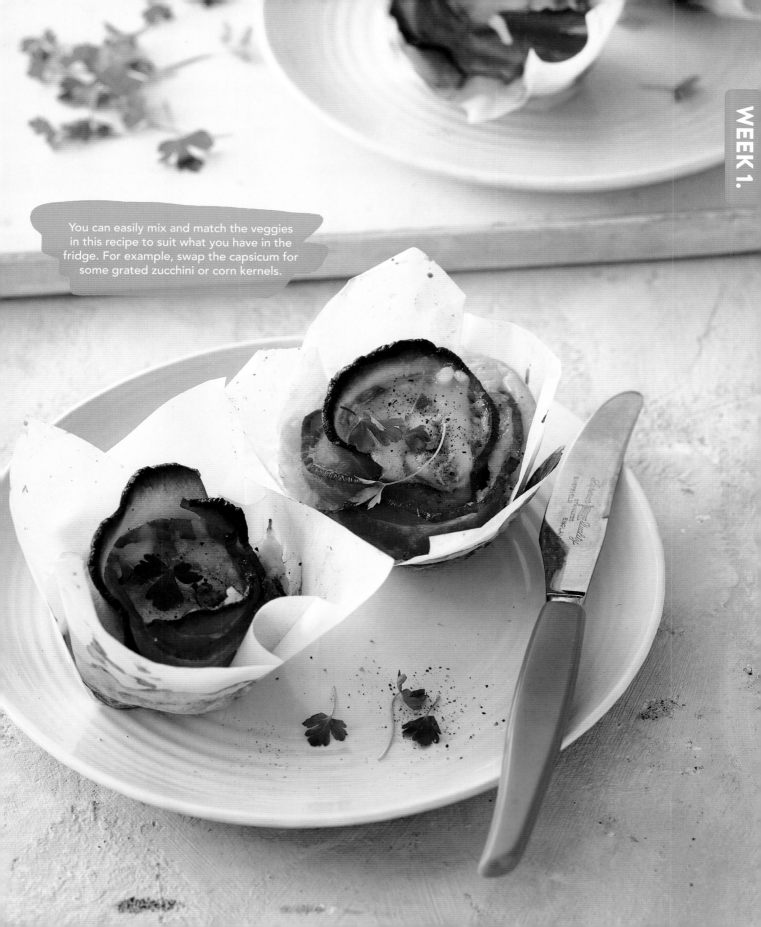

You can easily mix and match the veggies in this recipe to suit what you have in the fridge. For example, swap the capsicum for some grated zucchini or corn kernels.

EASY APPLE AND CINNAMON PORRIDGE

SERVES: 2   **PREPARATION TIME:** 5 MINUTES   **COOKING TIME:** 15 MINUTES

1 cup rolled oats

2 cups reduced-fat milk of choice

1 small apple, grated

½ teaspoon ground cinnamon

2 tablespoons chopped raw almonds

Combine the oats and milk in a small saucepan. Bring to the boil, then reduce the heat and simmer, stirring regularly, for 10 minutes or until smooth and creamy.

Stir through the apple and cinnamon.

Divide between two bowls and sprinkle with the chopped almonds to serve.

NUTRI DETAILS PER SERVE

337 cals/1415 kjs
Protein: 20 g
Fibre: 7.8 g
Total fat: 17.4 g
Sat fat: 3.4 g
Carbs: 23.8 g
Total sugar: 23.5 g
Free sugar: 0.0 g

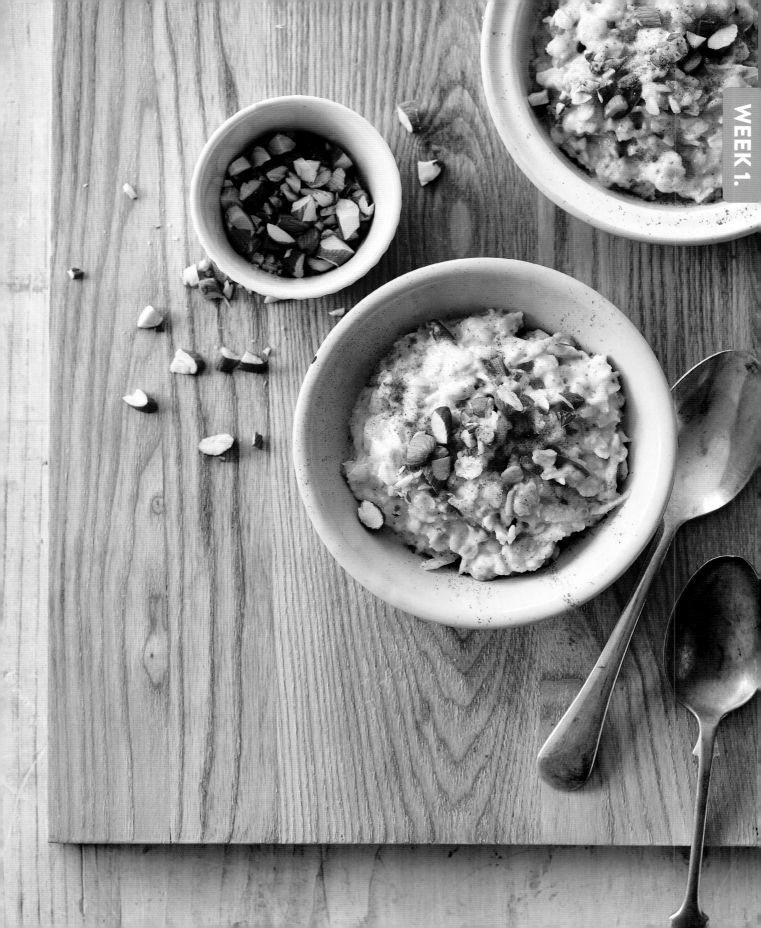

BREAKFAST QUINOA SALAD

SERVES: 2 **PREPARATION TIME:** 10 MINUTES, PLUS COOLING TIME **COOKING TIME:** 20 MINUTES

½ cup quinoa, rinsed

2 teaspoons pumpkin seeds

1 orange, peeled

1 teaspoon ground cinnamon, plus extra to serve

3 tablespoons raw almonds, chopped

3 tablespoons blueberries (fresh or frozen)

2 tablespoons reduced-fat Greek-style yoghurt

NUTRI DETAILS PER SERVE

362 cals/1514 kjs
Protein: 14 g
Fibre: 7.8 g
Total fat: 16.4 g
Sat fat: 1.7 g
Carbs: 35.8 g
Total sugar: 11.6 g
Free sugar: 0.0 g

Place the quinoa and 1 cup water in a small saucepan and bring to the boil. Reduce the heat and simmer, covered, for 20 minutes or until tender and most of the liquid has been absorbed. Fluff up with a fork, then set aside to cool.

Meanwhile, roast the pumpkin seeds in a dry frying pan over low heat, then set aside.

Cut the orange along either side of the white membranes to remove the segments, reserving any juice.

Add the reserved juice, cinnamon, pumpkin seeds, almonds and half the blueberries to the cooked quinoa and stir to combine.

Divide the quinoa mixture between two bowls, top with the remaining blueberries and orange segments, dollop with yoghurt and sprinkle with extra cinnamon to serve.

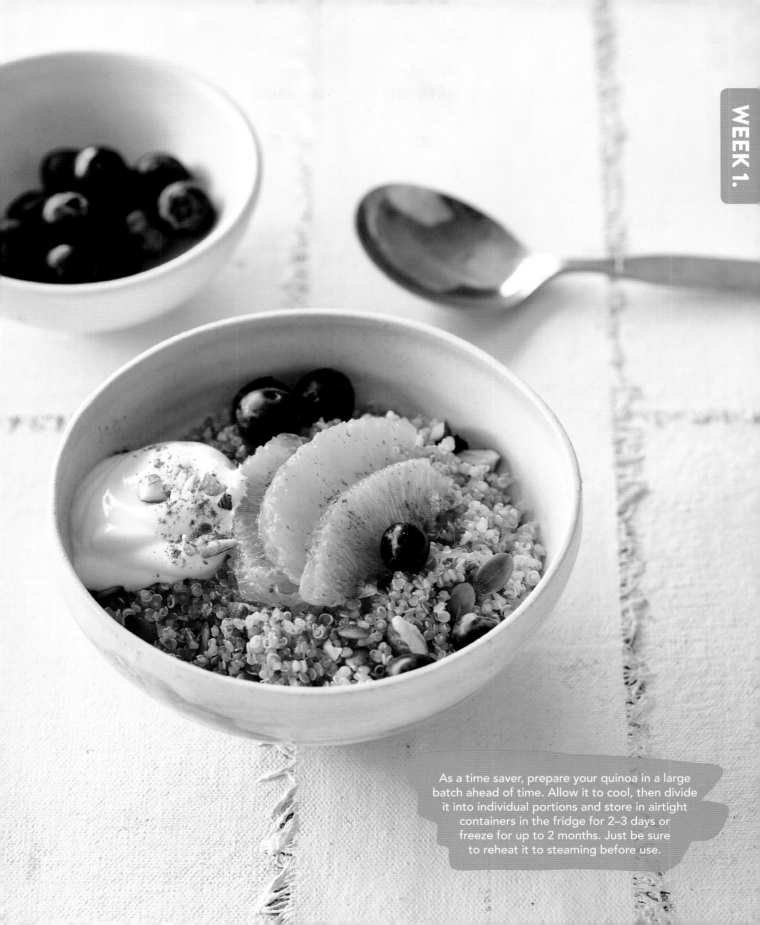

As a time saver, prepare your quinoa in a large batch ahead of time. Allow it to cool, then divide it into individual portions and store in airtight containers in the fridge for 2–3 days or freeze for up to 2 months. Just be sure to reheat it to steaming before use.

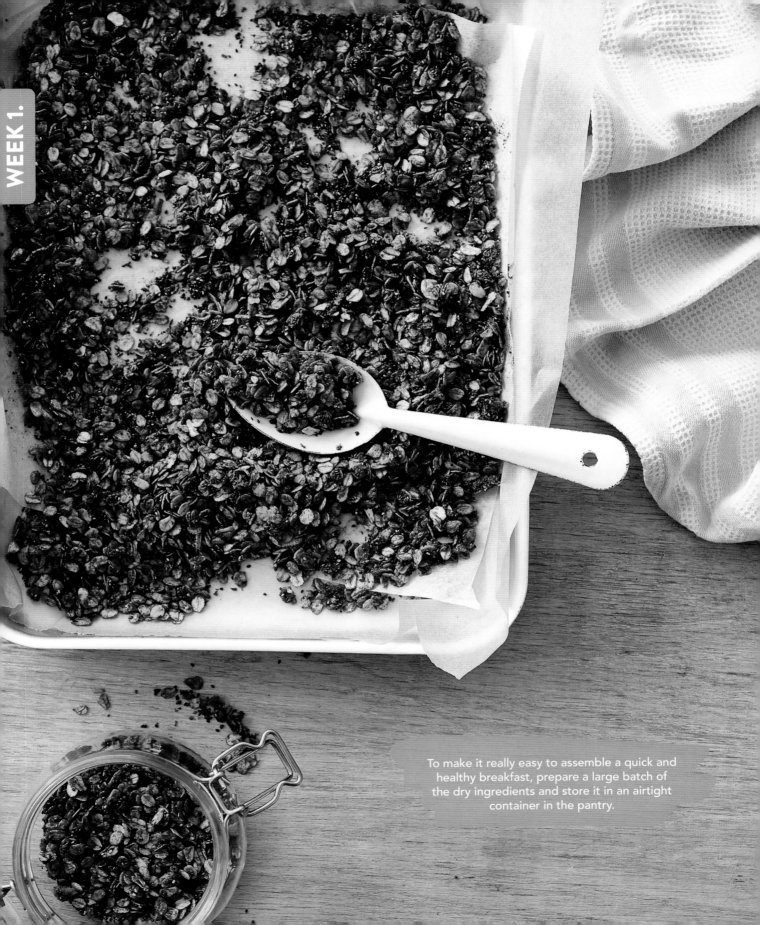

To make it really easy to assemble a quick and healthy breakfast, prepare a large batch of the dry ingredients and store it in an airtight container in the pantry.

CHOC–OAT GRANOLA

SERVES: 4 **PREPARATION TIME:** 5 MINUTES, PLUS COOLING TIME **COOKING TIME:** 15–20 MINUTES

1 cup rolled oats

⅓ cup desiccated coconut

3 tablespoons chia seeds

1 tablespoon cacao/cocoa powder

1 tablespoon coconut oil, melted

¼ teaspoon vanilla extract

1 tablespoon honey

2 cups reduced-fat milk of choice

NUTRI DETAILS PER SERVE

330 cals/1380 kjs
Protein: 10.6 g
Fibre: 8.2 g
Total fat: 17.8 g
Sat fat: 11 g
Carbs: 28 g
Total sugar: 13.2 g
Free sugar: 5.7 g

Preheat the oven to 180°C and line a baking tray with baking paper.

In a large bowl, stir together the oats, coconut, chia seeds and cacao/cocoa powder.

Combine the coconut oil, vanilla and honey and mix until smooth. Pour over the oat mixture and stir until well coated.

Spread the granola over the prepared tray and bake for 5 minutes. Stir, then bake for another 10–15 minutes or until lightly golden. Remove from the oven and cool completely without stirring.

Divide the granola among four bowls. Serve each portion with ½ cup milk for an easy, healthy breakfast.

Store any leftover granola in an airtight container in the pantry for 1–2 weeks.

BLT PITA MELT

SERVES: 2   **PREPARATION TIME:** 5 MINUTES   **COOKING TIME:** 15 MINUTES

---

3 lean bacon rashers, trimmed
1 tablespoon tomato passata
2 small wholemeal pita breads
1 tomato, sliced
3 tablespoons grated
  reduced-fat cheddar
30 g baby spinach leaves

NUTRI DETAILS PER SERVE

277 cals/1163 kjs
Protein: 22 g
Fibre: 4.6 g
Total fat: 8.8 g
Sat fat: 3.8 g
Carbs: 25 g
Total sugar: 2.9 g
Free sugar: 0.0 g

Preheat an overhead grill to high and line a baking tray with baking paper.

Place the bacon on the prepared tray and cook under the grill until crispy. Remove and slice the bacon.

Spread the passata evenly over the pita breads and place on the baking tray. Arrange the bacon and tomato on the breads and top with the grated cheese.

Cook under the grill for 8–10 minutes or until the cheese is melted and golden. Top with the baby spinach leaves and serve immediately.

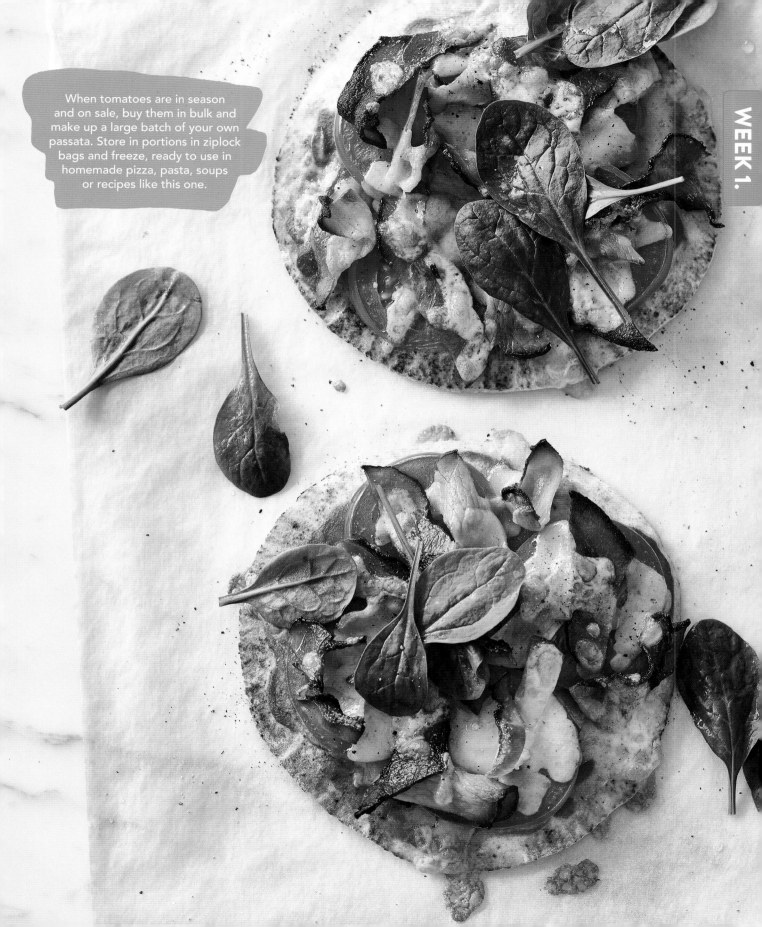

When tomatoes are in season and on sale, buy them in bulk and make up a large batch of your own passata. Store in portions in ziplock bags and freeze, ready to use in homemade pizza, pasta, soups or recipes like this one.

OAT AND CINNAMON PANCAKES

SERVES: 2   **PREPARATION TIME:** 5 MINUTES, PLUS SOAKING TIME   **COOKING TIME:** 10 MINUTES

½ cup rolled oats

½ cup reduced-fat milk of choice, plus extra if needed

2 free-range eggs, lightly beaten

½ cup plain wholemeal flour

½ teaspoon baking powder

1 teaspoon ground cinnamon

salt

olive oil spray

1 small banana, sliced

½ cup blueberries (fresh or frozen)

2 tablespoons reduced-fat Greek-style yoghurt

2 teaspoons pure maple syrup

Place the oats in a bowl, cover with the milk and set aside to soak for 10 minutes. Add the egg and stir to combine, then sift in the flour, baking powder, cinnamon and a pinch of salt and stir to form a smooth batter (add a little extra milk to thin if necessary).

Spray a large non-stick frying pan with olive oil and place over medium heat. Add 3 tablespoons of the batter for each pancake (you should be able to cook two pancakes at a time). Cook for 2 minutes or until bubbles start to form on the surface, then flip and cook for another 1–2 minutes or until golden. Repeat to make four pancakes in total.

Place two pancakes on each plate and serve topped with banana, blueberries, yoghurt and a drizzle of maple syrup.

NUTRI DETAILS PER SERVE

289 cals/1214 kjs
Protein: 13.5 g
Fibre: 3.5 g
Total fat: 7.3 g
Sat fat: 2.4 g
Carbs: 42.6 g
Total sugar: 4.4 g
Free sugar: 4 g

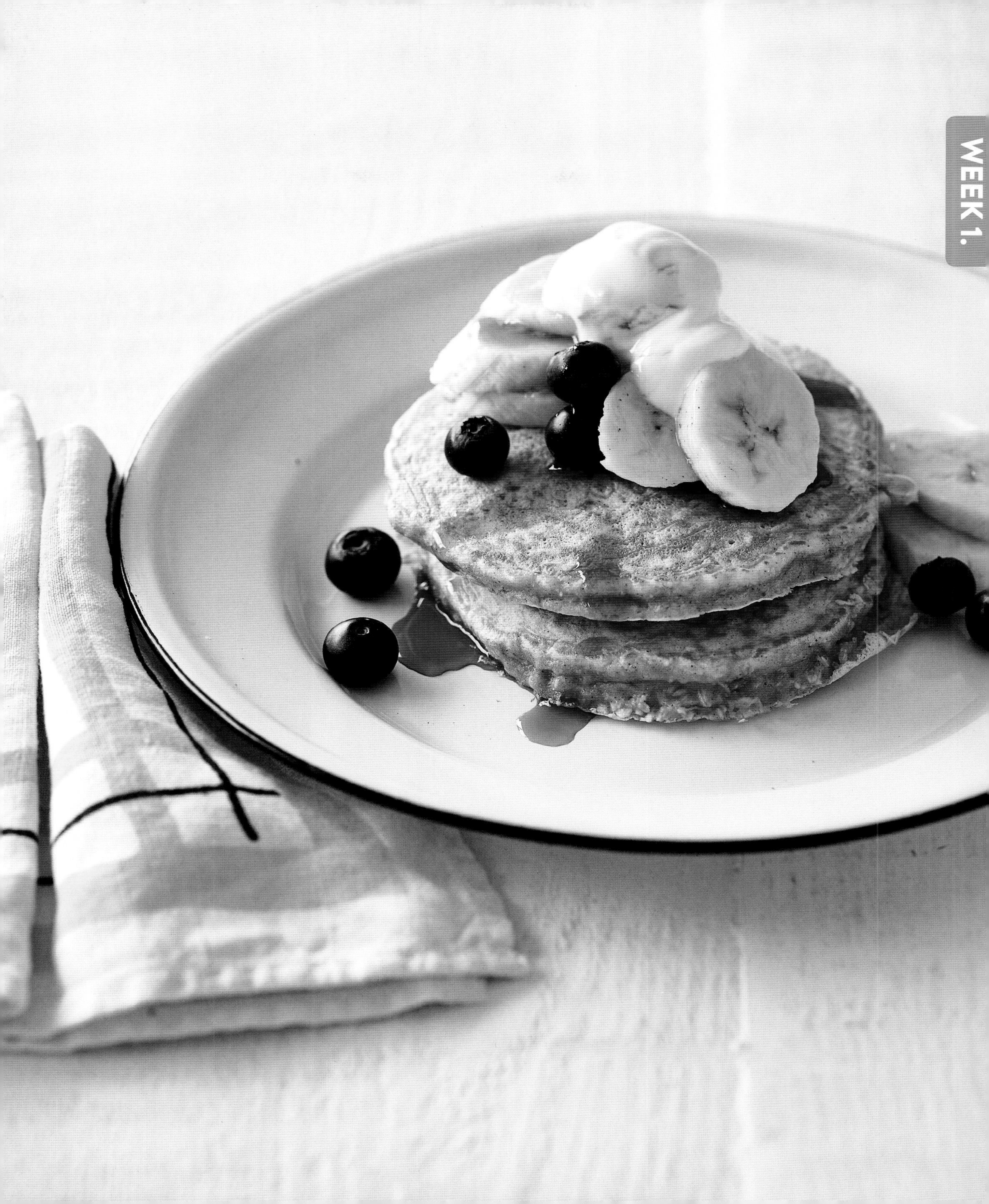

SALMON ROSTI

SERVES: 2   **PREPARATION TIME:** 10 MINUTES   **COOKING TIME:** 10 MINUTES

---

100 g tinned salmon in spring
water, drained

¼ red onion, finely chopped

1 free-range egg, lightly beaten

1 teaspoon wholegrain mustard

1 teaspoon dried dill

freshly ground black pepper

1 medium potato, peeled and
grated

1 tablespoon extra virgin
olive oil

2 tablespoons reduced-fat
Greek-style yoghurt

½ teaspoon baby capers, rinsed
and chopped

1 teaspoon lemon juice

fresh dill sprigs, to serve
(optional)

lemon wedges, to serve
(optional)

Combine the salmon, onion, egg, mustard, dill and pepper in a bowl. Add the potato and mix again briefly.

Heat the olive oil in a large frying pan over medium heat.

Divide the salmon mixture into four portions and form into rosti. Place the rosti in the frying pan and cook on each side for 3–4 minutes or until golden and the potato is cooked through.

Meanwhile, combine the yoghurt, capers and lemon juice in a bowl.

Serve two rosti on each plate, drizzled with the lemon yoghurt and with dill sprigs and lemon wedges, if desired.

NUTRI DETAILS PER SERVE

252 cals/1058 kjs
Protein: 16.6 g
Fibre: 1.6 g
Total fat: 14.9 g
Sat fat: 3 g
Carbs: 12 g
Total sugar: 2.3 g
Free sugar: 0.0 g

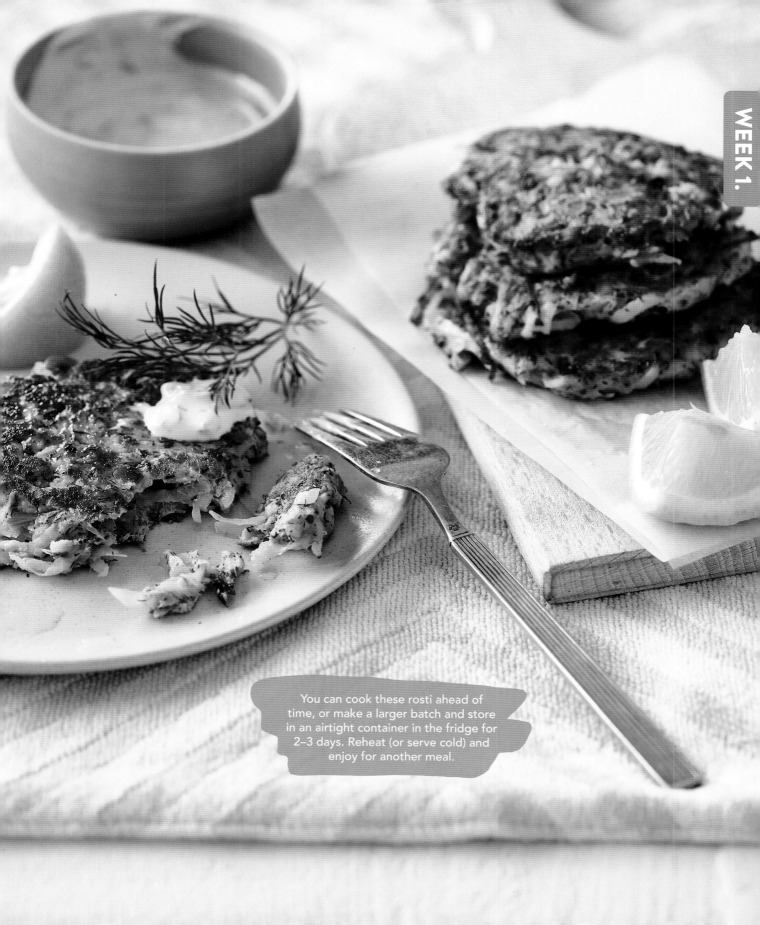

You can cook these rosti ahead of time, or make a larger batch and store in an airtight container in the fridge for 2–3 days. Reheat (or serve cold) and enjoy for another meal.

CHARGRILLED CAPSICUM, OLIVE AND CHEESE TOASTED SANDWICH

SERVES: 2   **PREPARATION TIME:** 5 MINUTES   **COOKING TIME:** 5 MINUTES

4 slices wholegrain or gluten-free bread of choice

50 g chargrilled capsicum strips, sliced (see tip, opposite), or use store-bought

2 tablespoons kalamata olives, pitted and diced

2 slices reduced-fat cheddar

20 g baby spinach leaves

Place two slices of bread on a board or plate and top with the capsicum strips, olives, cheese and spinach. Sandwich with the remaining slices of bread and toast in a preheated sandwich press.

If you don't have a sandwich press, toast as open sandwiches under a preheated overhead grill.

NUTRI DETAILS PER SERVE

297 cals/1246 kjs
Protein: 19 g
Fibre: 6.3 g
Total fat: 7.4 g
Sat fat: 2 g
Carbs: 35.4 g
Total sugar: 6.7 g
Free sugar: 0.0 g

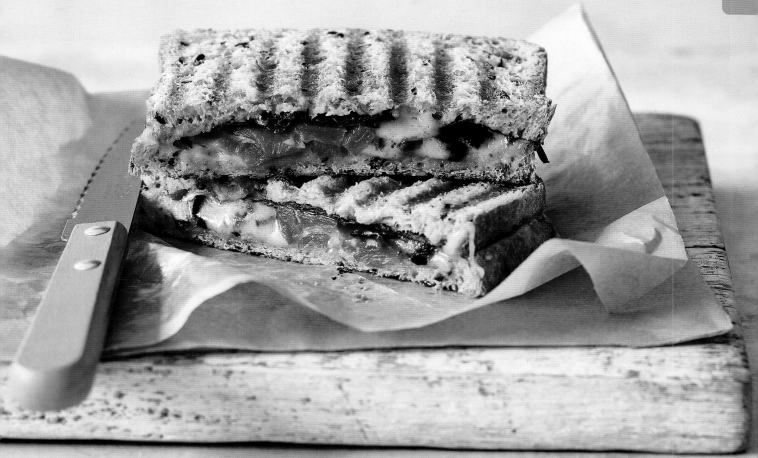

To make your own chargrilled capsicum strips, cut a capsicum in half, remove the seeds and place, skin-side down, on a preheated chargrill pan or barbecue plate. Cook for about 10 minutes or until the skin is black and blistered. Place the capsicum in a ziplock bag for 10 minutes to sweat, then peel off the skin. Transfer to a jar, add olive oil to cover and store in the fridge for up to a month.

BROWN RICE AND
RAW VEG POWER SALAD

SERVES: 2   **PREPARATION TIME:** 15 MINUTES, PLUS STANDING TIME   **COOKING TIME:** 45 MINUTES

½ cup brown rice

1 orange, peeled

1 tablespoon lemon juice

1 teaspoon finely grated lemon zest

1 teaspoon extra virgin olive oil

1 teaspoon pure maple syrup

200 g cauliflower, cut into small florets

2 medium carrots, grated

1 small zucchini, grated

2 celery stalks, finely sliced

2 spring onions, finely sliced

2 tablespoons dried cranberries

2 teaspoons pumpkin seeds

2 tablespoons small mint leaves

2 tablespoons crumbled reduced-fat feta

Bring 2 cups water to the boil in a medium saucepan, add the rice and simmer for 45 minutes or until tender. Drain and set aside to cool.

Cut the orange along either side of the white membranes to remove the segments, reserving any juice.

Combine the orange juice, lemon juice, lemon zest, olive oil and maple syrup in a large bowl. Add the cauliflower, carrot and zucchini and toss to coat with the juice mixture. Set aside for 5 minutes to develop the flavours.

Divide the orange segments, celery, spring onion, cranberries, rice and cauliflower mixture between two bowls and gently toss to combine. Sprinkle with the pumpkin seeds, mint and feta and serve.

NUTRI DETAILS PER SERVE

353 cals/1478 kjs
Protein: 12.5 g
Fibre: 8.3 g
Total fat: 8.9 g
Sat fat: 2.6 g
Carbs: 48.8 g
Total sugar: 17.9 g
Free sugar: 1.4 g

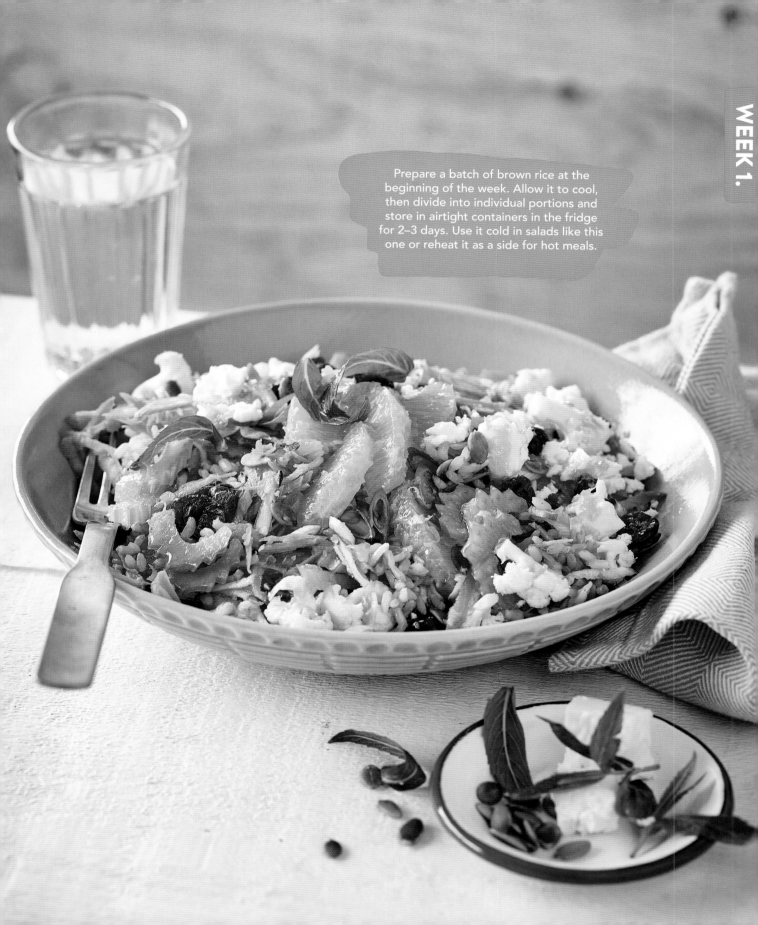

Prepare a batch of brown rice at the beginning of the week. Allow it to cool, then divide into individual portions and store in airtight containers in the fridge for 2–3 days. Use it cold in salads like this one or reheat it as a side for hot meals.

DETOX SOUP

SERVES: 4 **PREPARATION TIME:** 10 MINUTES **COOKING TIME:** 15 MINUTES

2 tablespoons extra virgin olive oil

2 garlic cloves, sliced

2 teaspoons grated ginger

1 teaspoon ground turmeric

salt

4 small zucchini, diced

1 litre salt-reduced vegetable stock

200 g broccoli florets

120 g kale leaves, shredded

2 tablespoons lime juice

1 bunch flat-leaf parsley leaves, chopped

2 teaspoons finely grated lime zest

Heat the olive oil in a large saucepan over medium–high heat. Add the garlic, ginger, turmeric and a pinch of salt and cook, stirring, for 2 minutes. Pour in ½ cup water.

Add the zucchini and cook for 3 minutes. Pour in the stock, then reduce the heat and simmer for 3 minutes. Add the broccoli florets, kale and lime juice and simmer for another 3–4 minutes or until all the vegetables are soft.

Remove the pan from the heat and add the parsley (reserving a few leaves for garnish). Use a stick blender or benchtop blender to blitz the soup until smooth.

Gently reheat the soup if required, then spoon into bowls and serve topped with lime zest and the extra parsley leaves.

NUTRI DETAILS PER SERVE

135 cals/567 kjs
Protein: 5 g
Fibre: 3.4 g
Total fat: 8.1 g
Sat fat: 1.2 g
Carbs: 14.1 g
Total sugar: 3.3 g
Free sugar: 0.0 g

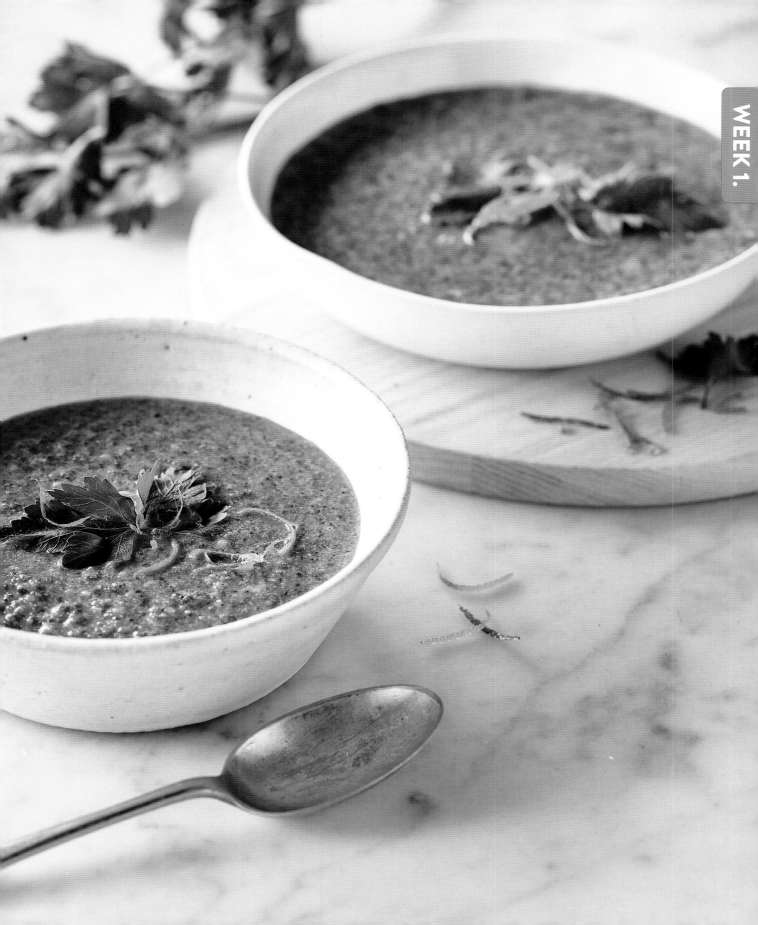

PROSCIUTTO, APPLE AND ROCKET SALAD

SERVES: 2   **PREPARATION TIME:** 10 MINUTES

120 g rocket leaves

2 small apples, sliced or cut into bite-sized pieces

120 g prosciutto, torn

3 tablespoons shaved parmesan

3 teaspoons balsamic vinegar

Divide the rocket between two bowls and add the apple and prosciutto.

Top with the shaved parmesan, drizzle with balsamic vinegar and serve.

NUTRI DETAILS PER SERVE

205 cals/861 kjs

Protein: 26 g

Fibre: 2.4 g

Total fat: 7 g

Sat fat: 6.2 g

Carbs: 9.9 g

Total sugar: 9.9 g

Free sugar: 0.0 g

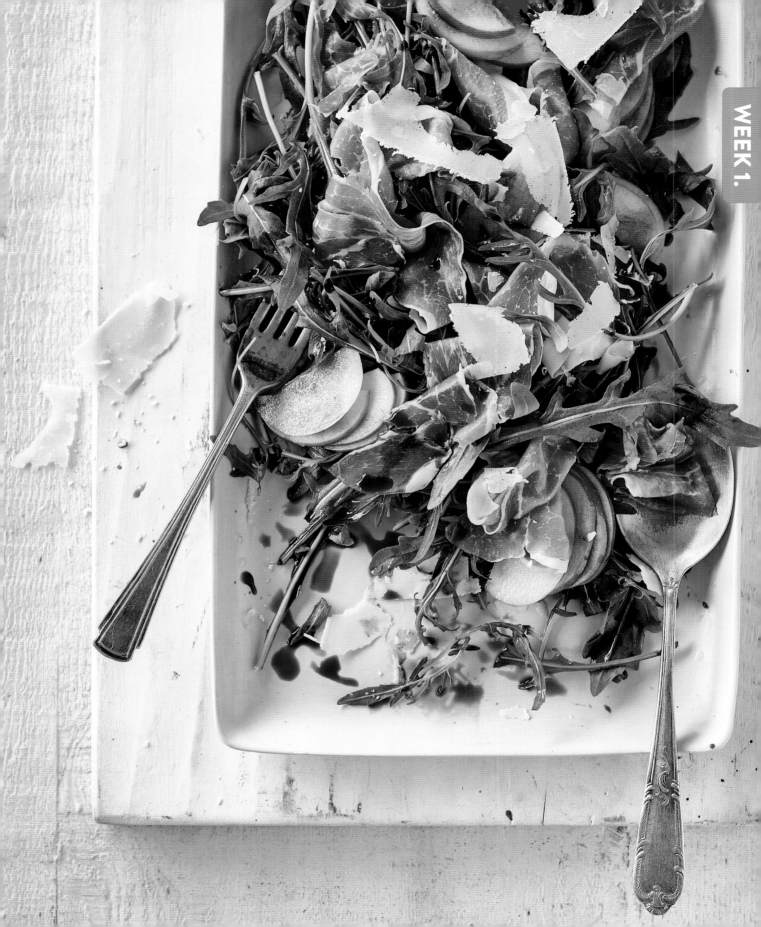

Make a large batch of fritters, let them cool and freeze for up to a month, then all you need to do is thaw and reheat them for another meal.

CORN AND QUINOA FRITTERS

SERVES: 2   **PREPARATION TIME:** 10 MINUTES, PLUS COOLING TIME   **COOKING TIME:** 25 MINUTES

½ cup quinoa, rinsed

½ cup corn kernels (fresh or tinned)

1 tablespoon plain wholemeal flour

2 free-range eggs, lightly beaten

¼ red onion, diced

2 teaspoons grated parmesan

salt and freshly ground black pepper

1 tablespoon coconut oil

2 teaspoons sweet chilli sauce

2 spring onions, sliced

Place the quinoa and 1 cup water in a small saucepan and bring to the boil. Reduce the heat and simmer, covered, for 15 minutes or until tender and most of the liquid has been absorbed. Fluff up with a fork, then set aside to cool.

Combine the cooled quinoa, corn, flour, egg, red onion, half the parmesan and a pinch of salt and pepper in a bowl.

Melt the coconut oil in a frying pan over medium–high heat. Divide the batter into six portions, then add them to the pan, flattening them slightly. Cook for 2–3 minutes on each side or until golden and cooked through. Remove and drain on paper towel.

Place three fritters on each plate and drizzle with the sweet chilli sauce. Top with the spring onion and remaining parmesan and serve.

NUTRI DETAILS PER SERVE

348 cals/1465 kjs
Protein: 15.5 g
Fibre: 5.3 g
Total fat: 14.2 g
Sat fat: 9.2 g
Carbs: 40.9 g
Total sugar: 2 g
Free sugar: 0.7 g

EASY PIZZA WRAPS

SERVES: 2   **PREPARATION TIME:** 10 MINUTES   **COOKING TIME:** 5 MINUTES

---

130 g reduced-fat ricotta

4 wholemeal mountain bread wraps

6 slices lean smoked ham

2 tablespoons kalamata olives, pitted and chopped

1 tomato, sliced

freshly ground black pepper

2 cups mixed leaf salad, to serve

Spread the ricotta evenly over the wraps, then top with the ham, olives and tomato slices. Season with pepper and roll up to enclose the filling.

Place in a preheated sandwich press and toast for 1–2 minutes or until warmed through. If you don't have a sandwich press, cook the wraps under a preheated overhead grill for 1–2 minutes each side.

Place two wraps on each plate and serve immediately with salad leaves.

NUTRI DETAILS PER SERVE

323 cals/1355 kjs
Protein: 25.5 g
Fibre: 4.8 g
Total fat: 8.8 g
Sat fat: 4.6 g
Carbs: 32.9 g
Total sugar: 10.8 g
Free sugar: 0.0 g

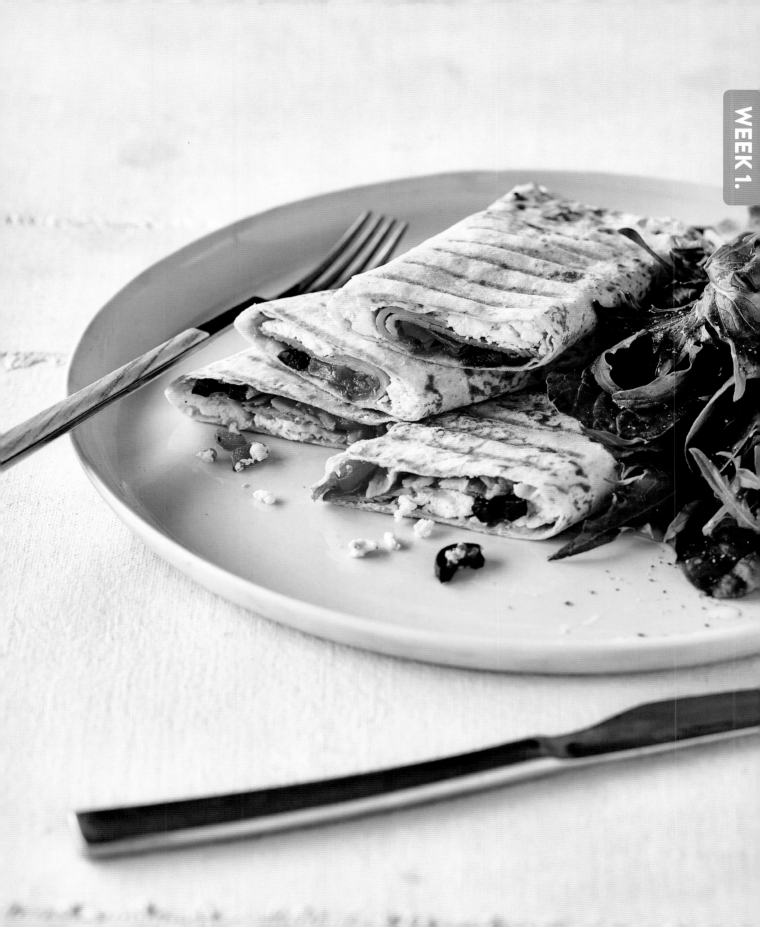

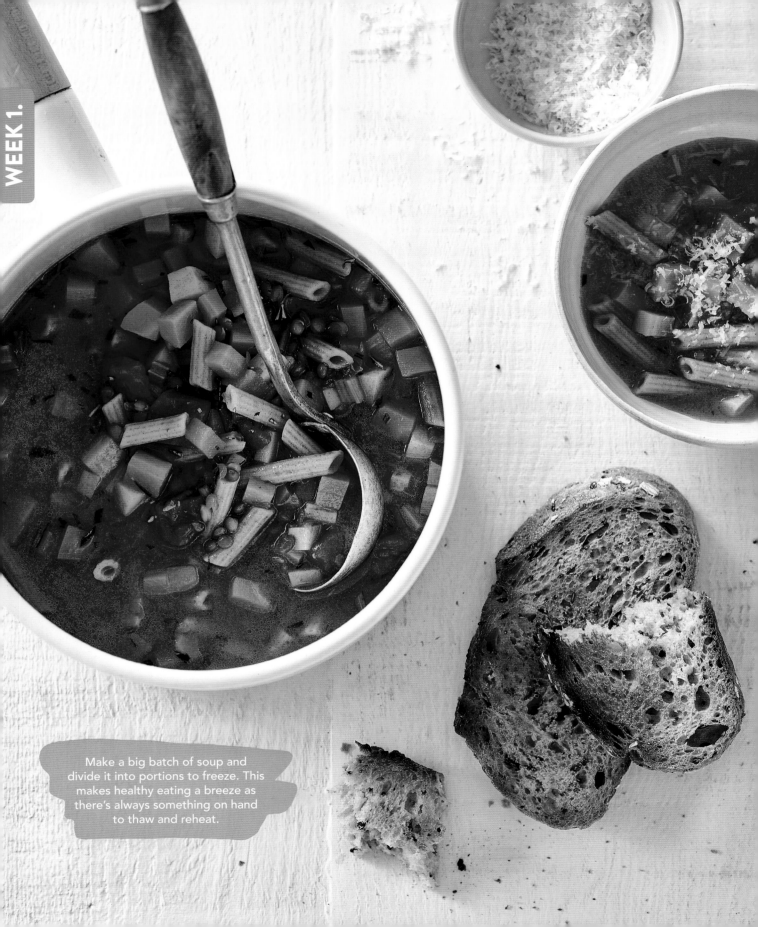

Make a big batch of soup and divide it into portions to freeze. This makes healthy eating a breeze as there's always something on hand to thaw and reheat.

AUTUMN MINESTRONE

SERVES: 2   PREPARATION TIME: 10 MINUTES   COOKING TIME: 25 MINUTES

1 teaspoon extra virgin olive oil

1 garlic clove, finely chopped

1 medium carrot, diced

½ celery stalk, diced

½ medium potato, diced

200 g tinned diced tomatoes

1 cup salt-reduced vegetable stock, plus extra if needed

2 tablespoons wholemeal pasta (any shape)

2 tablespoons tinned lentils, rinsed and drained

½ teaspoon fresh rosemary, chopped, plus extra to garnish

2 slices wholegrain or gluten-free bread of choice

2 tablespoons grated parmesan

Heat the olive oil in a medium saucepan over medium heat. Add the garlic and saute for 30–60 seconds or until fragrant. Add the carrot, celery and potato and toss to coat with the oil and garlic, then cook for a further 1–2 minutes.

Add the tinned tomatoes, stock, pasta, lentils and rosemary. Bring the mixture to the boil, then reduce the heat and simmer for 15–20 minutes or until the pasta is cooked through. Add a little more stock if the soup is getting too thick.

Just before you are ready to serve, toast the bread. Ladle the soup into two bowls, sprinkle with the parmesan and extra rosemary, and serve with the hot toast.

NUTRI DETAILS PER SERVE

333 cals/1397 kjs
Protein: 15 g
Fibre: 7.5 g
Total fat: 10.5 g
Sat fat: 2.8 g
Carbs: 40 g
Total sugar: 6.7 g
Free sugar: 0.0 g

COCONUT LAMB WITH CAULIFLOWER RICE

SERVES: 4   PREPARATION TIME: 15 MINUTES   COOKING TIME: 35 MINUTES

2 tablespoons coconut oil

4 garlic cloves, crushed

400 g lean lamb steak, cut into 2 cm cubes

2 cups reduced-fat coconut milk

800 g cauliflower, cut into florets

salt and freshly ground black pepper

2 tomatoes, diced

1 small zucchini, halved lengthways then sliced

⅓ cup coriander leaves

Melt 1 tablespoon of the coconut oil in a saucepan over medium heat, add the garlic and cook for 1 minute. Add the lamb and brown on all sides. Pour in the coconut milk, then reduce the heat to low and simmer for 25–30 minutes or until the lamb is tender.

While the lamb is cooking, place the cauliflower in a food processor and blitz until it resembles rice.

Melt the remaining coconut oil in a frying pan over medium–high heat, add the cauliflower rice and season with salt and pepper. Stir well and cook for 4–5 minutes or until the cauliflower is tender.

About 5 minutes before the lamb is ready, add the tomato and zucchini and stir to combine. Cook for a few minutes until the veggies are tender.

Divide the coconut rice among four plates and spoon the coconut lamb and vegetables over the top. Sprinkle with the coriander and serve.

NUTRI DETAILS PER SERVE

397 cals/1669 kjs
Protein: 28.4 g
Fibre: 5.3 g
Total fat: 25 g
Sat fat: 19.6 g
Carbs: 12.1 g
Total sugar: 10.2 g
Free sugar: 0.0 g

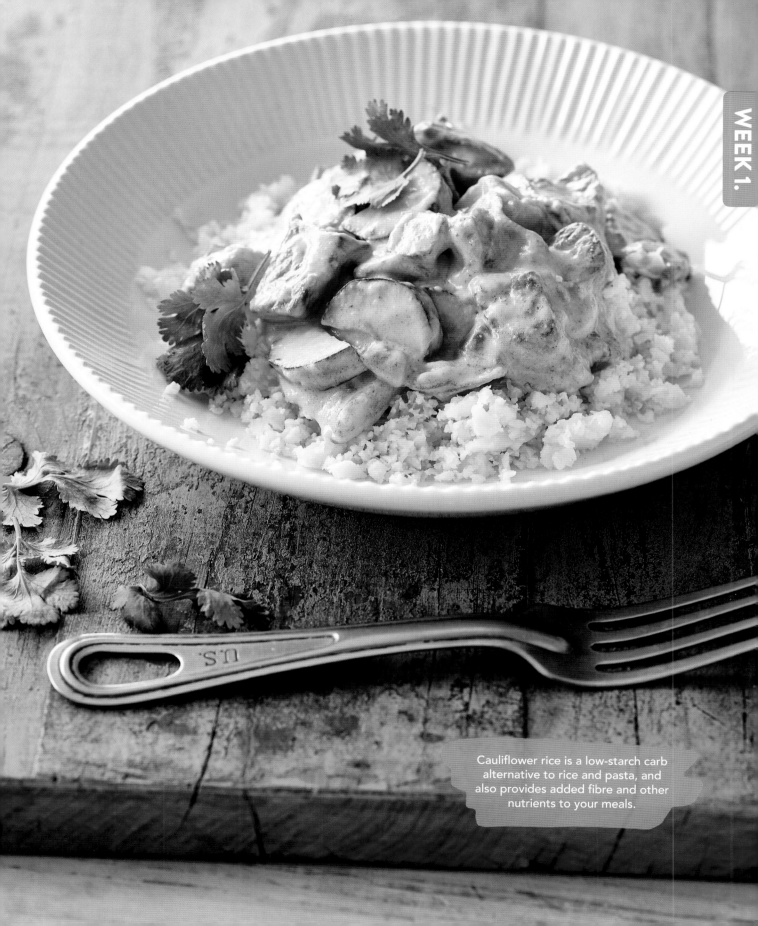

Cauliflower rice is a low-starch carb alternative to rice and pasta, and also provides added fibre and other nutrients to your meals.

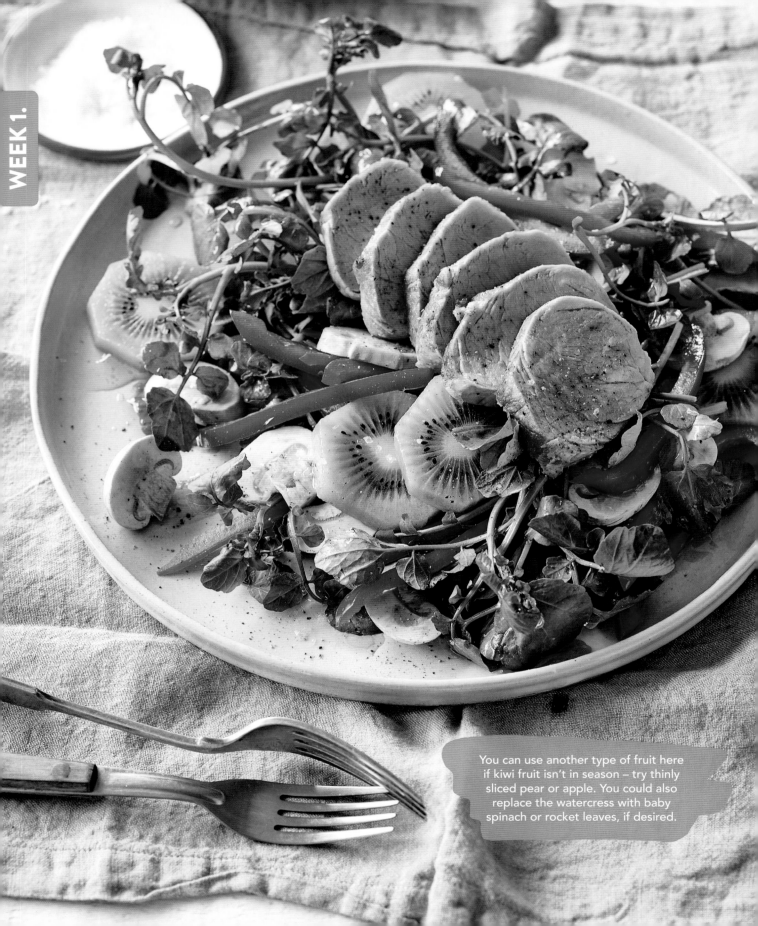

You can use another type of fruit here if kiwi fruit isn't in season – try thinly sliced pear or apple. You could also replace the watercress with baby spinach or rocket leaves, if desired.

PORK WITH KIWI FRUIT AND WATERCRESS SALAD

SERVES: 4   **PREPARATION TIME:** 10 MINUTES   **COOKING TIME:** 10 MINUTES

cooking oil spray

400 g pork fillet, cut into
1 cm slices

300 g mushrooms, sliced

2 kiwi fruit, peeled and sliced

2 red capsicums, seeds
removed, finely sliced

70 g watercress

2 tablespoons red wine vinegar

1 tablespoon extra virgin
olive oil

salt and freshly ground black
pepper

Lightly spray a frying pan with cooking oil spray and place over medium–high heat. Add the pork and cook for 4–5 minutes each side or until cooked through. Remove and set aside to rest.

In a bowl combine the mushroom, kiwi fruit, capsicum, watercress, vinegar and olive oil, and season to taste with salt and pepper.

Divide the salad among four bowls. Arrange the pork on top of the salad and serve.

NUTRI DETAILS PER SERVE

418 cals/1755 kjs
Protein: 34.6 g
Fibre: 4.9 g
Total fat: 23.2 g
Sat fat: 6.1 g
Carbs: 19.8 g
Total sugar: 11.7 g
Free sugar: 0.0 g

CHICKEN NOODLE STIR-FRY

SERVES: 4   **PREPARATION TIME:** 15 MINUTES, PLUS SOAKING TIME   **COOKING TIME:** 10 MINUTES

200 g rice vermicelli noodles

1 tablespoon coconut oil

400 g chicken breast fillets, cut into 1 cm-thick strips

1 tablespoon finely grated ginger

400 g broccoli, cut into florets

2 heads bok choy, chopped

150 g mushrooms, sliced

2 tablespoons salt-reduced soy sauce

½ lemon

NUTRI DETAILS PER SERVE

282 cals/1186 kjs
Protein: 29.9 g
Fibre: 5.7 g
Total fat: 11 g
Sat fat: 6 g
Carbs: 12.5 g
Total sugar: 1.1 g
Free sugar: 0.0 g

Place the vermicelli noodles in a heatproof bowl and cover with boiling water. Allow to soak for 10 minutes or until the noodles are tender. Drain well.

Meanwhile, melt the coconut oil in a wok or frying pan over medium–high heat. Add the chicken and ginger and cook for 1–2 minutes or until the chicken is brown all over. Add the broccoli and cook for 1–2 minutes, then add the bok choy and mushrooms and cook for another minute. Pour in the soy sauce and toss well.

Add the noodles to the pan and toss to combine.

Divide the stir-fry among four bowls, finish with a squeeze of lemon juice and serve immediately.

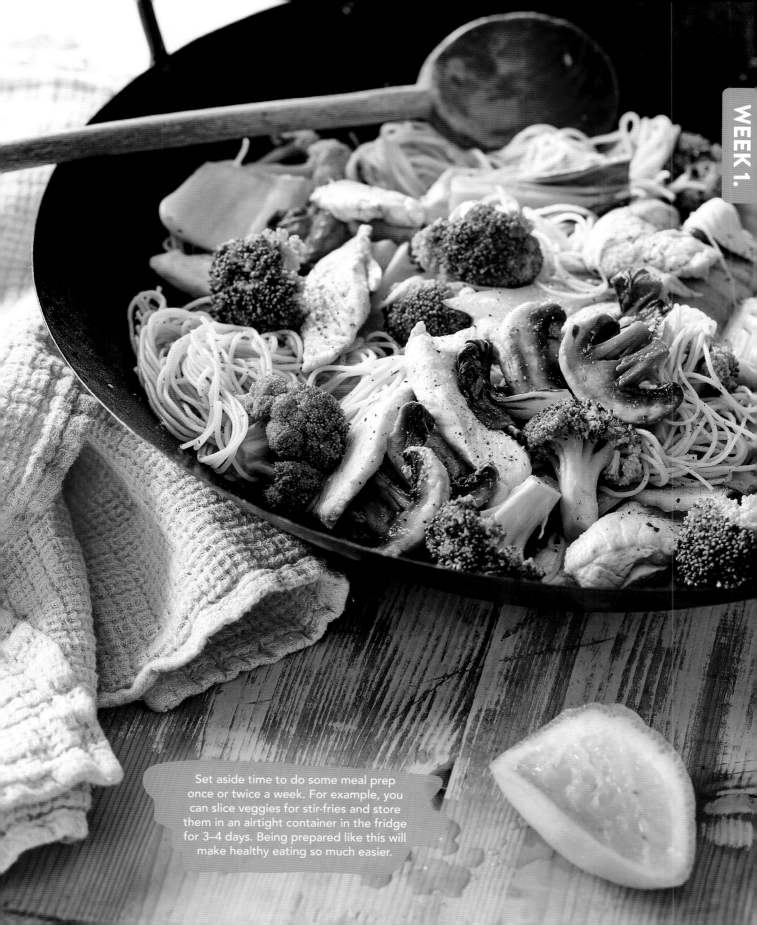

Set aside time to do some meal prep once or twice a week. For example, you can slice veggies for stir-fries and store them in an airtight container in the fridge for 3–4 days. Being prepared like this will make healthy eating so much easier.

MEXICAN LASAGNE

SERVES: 4   **PREPARATION TIME:** 15 MINUTES   **COOKING TIME:** 1 HOUR

2 brown onions, finely diced

400 g lean beef mince

2 medium carrots, grated

1 red capsicum, seeds removed, finely chopped

1 × 400 g tin kidney beans, drained and rinsed

1 × 400 g tin diced tomatoes

1 tablespoon salt-reduced taco seasoning

cooking oil spray

5 wholemeal tortillas

½ cup reduced-fat Greek-style yoghurt

100 g reduced-fat cheddar, grated

NUTRI DETAILS PER SERVE

483 cals/2026 kjs
Protein: 40 g
Fibre: 10.7 g
Total fat: 16.2 g
Sat fat: 7.4 g
Carbs: 38.4 g
Total sugar: 13.4 g
Free sugar: 0.0 g

Preheat the oven to 180°C.

Heat a non-stick frying pan over medium–high heat. Add the onion and cook for a couple of minutes, then add 1 tablespoon water (this eliminates the need to add any oil) and cook for 5 minutes or until the onion is soft and translucent and the water has evaporated.

Increase the heat to high. Add the mince and cook, breaking up any lumps with the back of a wooden spoon, until the mince is nicely browned. Add the carrot, capsicum, kidney beans, diced tomatoes and taco seasoning and stir well. Reduce the heat and simmer for 10–15 minutes or until the mixture has thickened.

Lightly spray a round baking dish with cooking oil spray.

Place a tortilla on the base of the dish and spoon over some of the meat mixture. Continue layering with the remaining tortillas and meat mixture, finishing with a tortilla. Spread the yoghurt over the top tortilla, then sprinkle evenly with the cheese. Bake for 30–40 minutes or until golden brown.

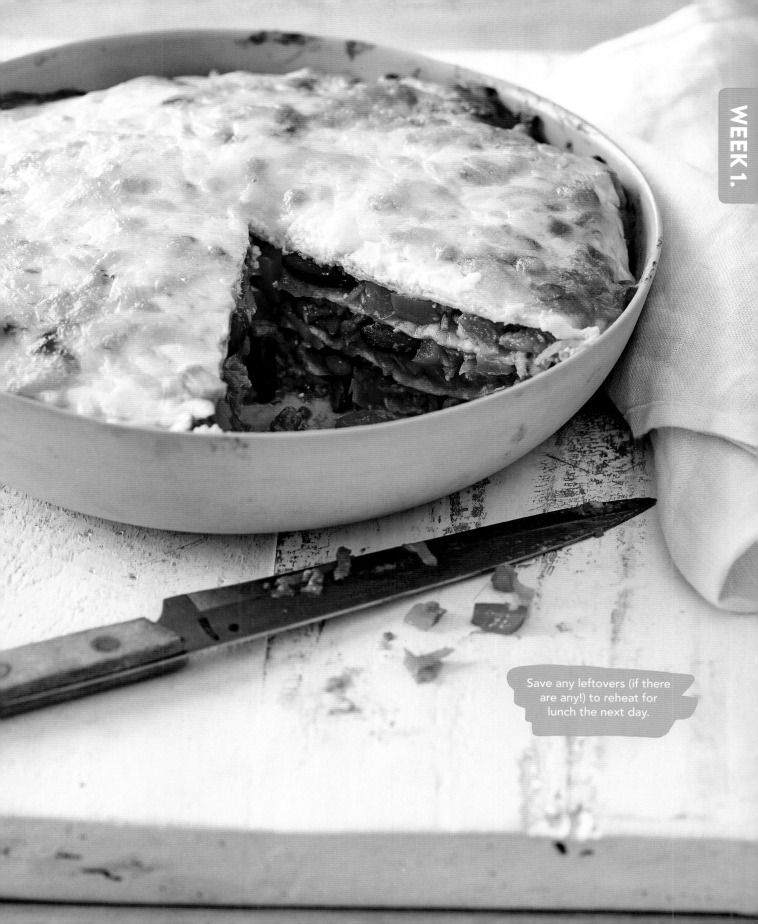

Save any leftovers (if there are any!) to reheat for lunch the next day.

FISH AND VEGGIE KEBABS

SERVES: 4   **PREPARATION TIME:** 15 MINUTES, PLUS SOAKING TIME   **COOKING TIME:** 10 MINUTES

4 garlic cloves, crushed

2 tablespoons extra virgin olive oil

⅓ cup lemon juice

⅓ cup finely chopped flat-leaf parsley leaves

600 g white fish fillet of choice, skin and bones removed, cut into 3–4 cm chunks

2 small zucchini, cut into chunks

2 red capsicums, seeds removed, cut into chunks

1 red onion, cut into chunks

lemon wedges, to serve (optional)

You will need eight skewers for this recipe. If you are using wooden skewers, soak them in water for 30 minutes before use so they don't burn during cooking.

Combine the garlic, olive oil, lemon juice and parsley in a bowl.

Thread the fish and vegetable chunks evenly onto the skewers, then brush all over with the parsley marinade.

Heat a large frying pan over medium–high heat and cook the kebabs for 3–4 minutes on each side or until the fish is cooked through and the vegetables are tender. Serve immediately, with lemon wedges if desired.

NUTRI DETAILS PER SERVE

286 cals/1202 kjs
Protein: 32.6 g
Fibre: 3.9 g
Total fat: 11.8 g
Sat fat: 1 g
Carbs: 9.9 g
Total sugar: 8.1 g
Free sugar: 0.0 g

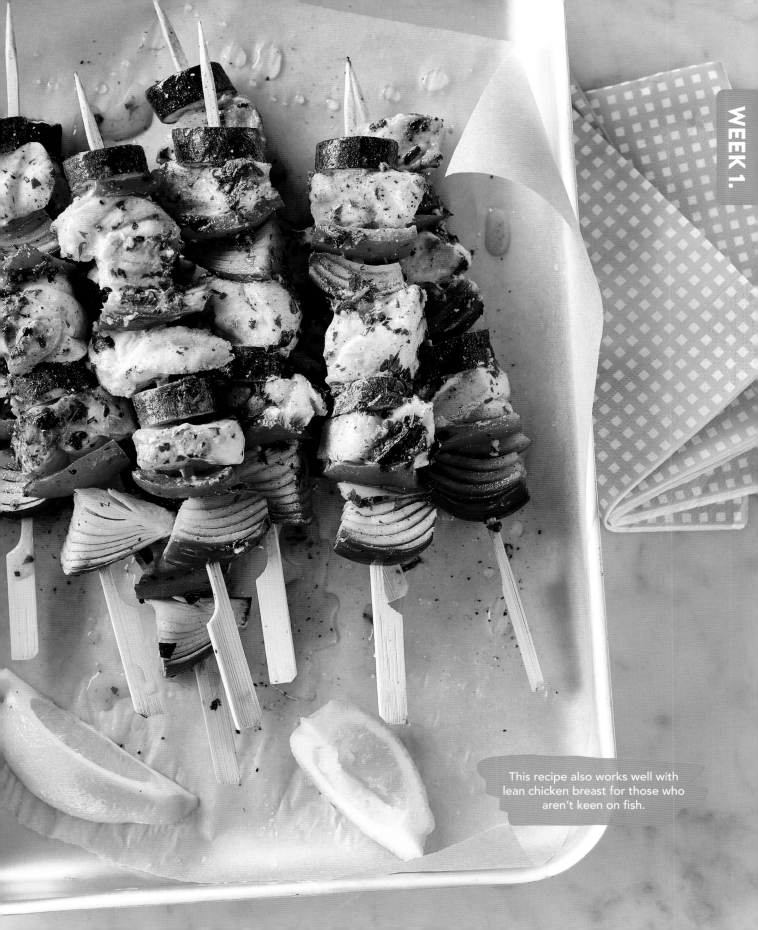

This recipe also works well with lean chicken breast for those who aren't keen on fish.

Zoodles make a great low-starch carbohydrate alternative to pasta and noodles. If other members of your family love pasta you could always serve your dish with the zoodles and offer spaghetti for everyone else.

ZOODLES WITH HALOUMI AND ROASTED VEGETABLES

SERVES: 4   PREPARATION TIME: 15 MINUTES   COOKING TIME: 30 MINUTES

2 red capsicums, seeds removed, roughly chopped

4 flat mushrooms, cut into large pieces

4 small roma tomatoes, halved

1 brown onion, roughly chopped

4 garlic cloves, finely chopped

2 teaspoons fresh thyme leaves

¼ cup extra virgin olive oil

160 g haloumi, cut into 8 slices

4 small zucchini

NUTRI DETAILS PER SERVE

272 cals/1143 kjs
Protein: 11.9 g
Fibre: 3.7 g
Total fat: 21.5 g
Sat fat: 6.4 g
Carbs: 6.5 g
Total sugar: 5.9 g
Free sugar: 0.0 g

Preheat the oven to 200°C and line a baking tray with baking paper.

Place the capsicum, mushroom, tomato, onion, garlic, thyme and 2 tablespoons of the olive oil in a bowl and gently toss to combine. Spread out the vegetables on the prepared tray and roast for 25–30 minutes or until tender.

Shortly before the vegetables are ready, heat the remaining olive oil in a frying pan over medium–high heat. Add the haloumi slices and cook for 1–2 minutes each side or until golden and tender.

Meanwhile, use a spiraliser or vegetable peeler to slice the zucchini into long noodles (zoodles).

When the vegetables are almost ready, blanch the zoodles in a saucepan of boiling water for 1 minute or until just tender.

Toss the roasted vegetables with the zoodles, then divide among four plates. Top with the warm haloumi and serve.

LOADED SWEET POTATO FRIES

SERVES: 4   **PREPARATION TIME:** 15 MINUTES   **COOKING TIME:** 35 MINUTES

4 small sweet potatoes, cut into wide chips

2 tablespoons extra virgin olive oil

200 g tinned kidney beans, drained and rinsed

1 red onion, diced

⅓ cup grated reduced-fat cheddar

2 medium avocados, diced

⅓ cup coriander leaves

NUTRI DETAILS PER SERVE

397 cals/1670 kjs
Protein: 16.5 g
Fibre: 7.5 g
Total fat: 22.7 g
Sat fat: 5 g
Carbs: 29 g
Total sugar: 10.5 g
Free sugar: 0.0 g

Preheat the oven to 180°C and line a baking tray with baking paper.

Coat the sweet potato chips with 1 tablespoon of the olive oil and spread over the prepared tray. Bake for 25–30 minutes or until roasted and tender, turning halfway through cooking.

Meanwhile, heat the remaining olive oil in a frying pan over medium–high heat, add the kidney beans and onion and cook for 2–3 minutes or until the onion has softened.

Remove the sweet potato fries from the oven and transfer to an ovenproof serving dish. Top with the bean mixture and grated cheese, then return to the oven for 4–5 minutes or until the cheese has melted.

Divide the fries among four plates, top with the avocado and coriander and serve.

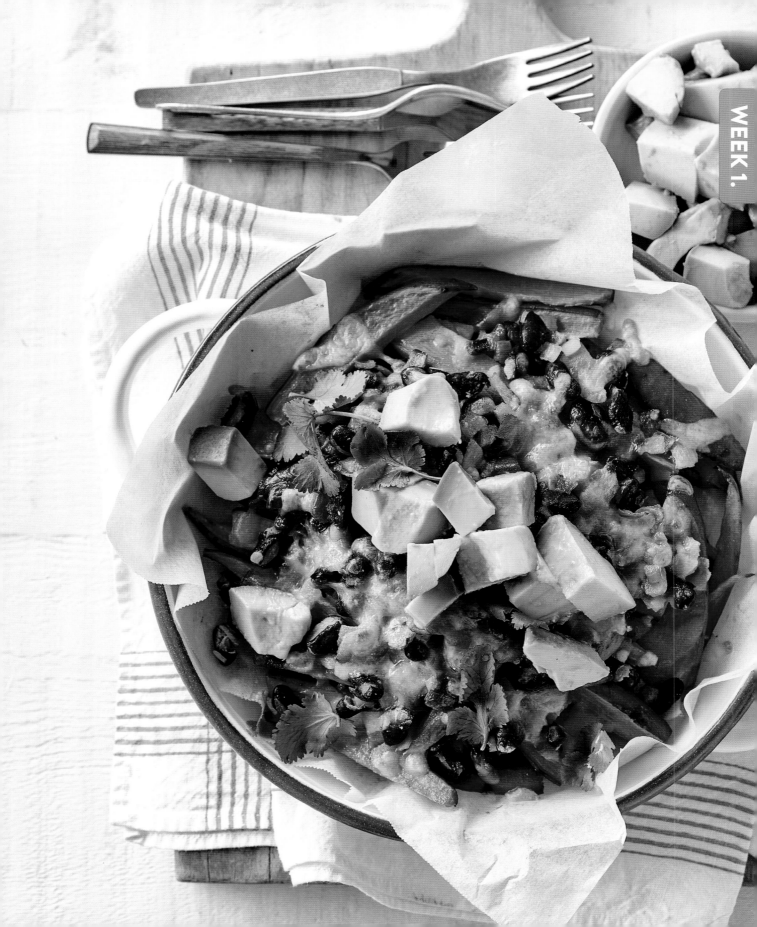

MEXICAN LAYERED DIP

SERVES: 4   **PREPARATION TIME:** 10 MINUTES   **COOKING TIME:** 10 MINUTES

240 g tinned red kidney beans, drained and rinsed
salt and freshly ground black pepper
2 spring onions, finely sliced
1 medium avocado
½ teaspoon dried chilli flakes
1 tablespoon lime juice
⅓ cup reduced-fat Greek-style yoghurt
2 tomatoes, chopped
1 tablespoon grated reduced-fat cheddar
4 hard taco shells

Preheat the oven to 160°C.

Place the kidney beans in a bowl and lightly mash with a fork. Mix with 2 tablespoons water to loosen and season with salt and pepper, then stir through the spring onion.

Mash the avocado, chilli flakes and lime juice in a separate bowl until smooth and well combined.

Divide the bean mixture among four small dishes. Top each dish with an even amount of yoghurt, mashed avocado, tomato and grated cheese.

Heat the taco shells in the oven for 6–7 minutes, then break them into chips for dipping.

Divide the chips into four portions and serve with the individual bowls of dip. Any leftover dip will keep, covered, in the fridge for 3–4 days.

NUTRI DETAILS PER SERVE

208 cals/873 kjs
Protein: 10.9 g
Fibre: 6.4 g
Total fat: 9.4 g
Sat fat: 3.2 g
Carbs: 17.5 g
Total sugar: 4.9 g
Free sugar: 0.0 g

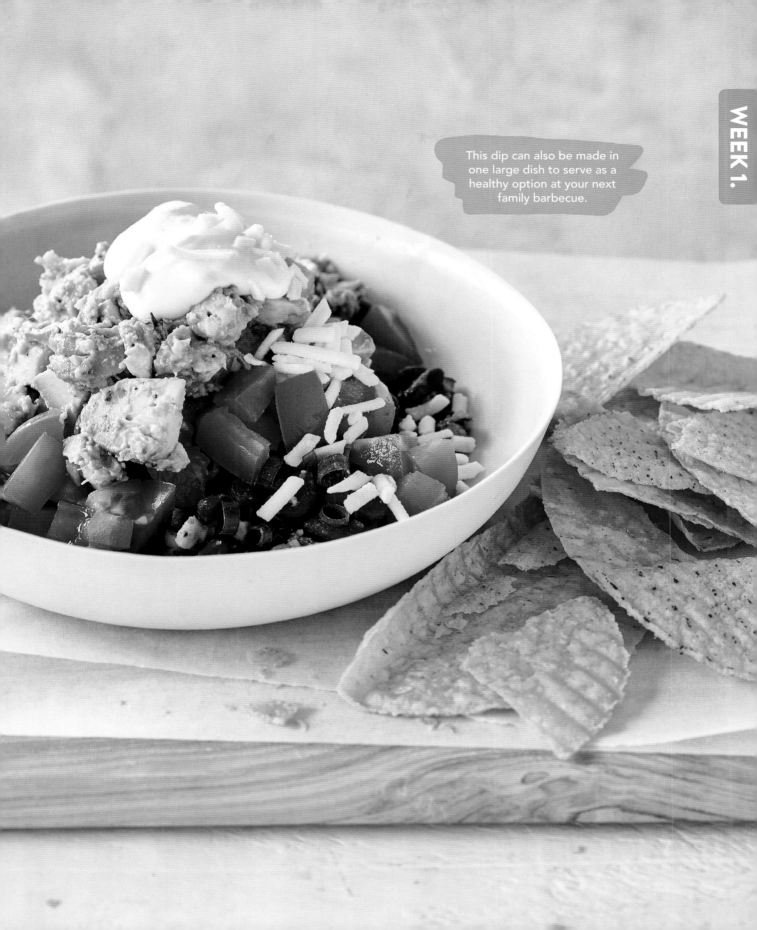

This dip can also be made in one large dish to serve as a healthy option at your next family barbecue.

PEANUT BUTTER AND CHOCOLATE COOKIES

SERVES: 5   **PREPARATION TIME:** 10 MINUTES, PLUS STANDING AND CHILLING TIME
COOKING TIME: 15 MINUTES

½ teaspoon chia seeds

30 g butter, at room temperature

2 tablespoons coconut sugar

1 ½ tablespoons peanut butter

⅓ cup plain wholemeal flour

½ teaspoon baking powder

3 teaspoons cacao/cocoa powder

NUTRI DETAILS PER SERVE

147 cals/618 kjs
Protein: 3.5 g
Fibre: 1.4 g
Total fat: 9.4 g
Sat fat: 4 g
Carbs: 11.9 g
Total sugar: 5 g
Free sugar: 4.6 g

Soak the chia seeds in 1 teaspoon water for 10 minutes so they plump up.

Cream the butter and coconut sugar with electric beaters. Add the peanut butter and chia gel and mix them in, then add the flour, baking powder and cacao/cocao powder and mix until well combined and a dough forms.

Roll the dough into a log and wrap in plastic wrap, then place in the fridge to firm for 20–30 minutes.

Preheat the oven to 180°C and line a baking tray with baking paper.

Cut the cookie dough log into five even rounds and place them on the prepared tray, leaving plenty of room for spreading. Bake for 10–15 minutes or until golden. Cool on the tray for a few minutes, then transfer the cookies to a wire rack to cool completely. Store in an airtight container in the pantry for up to a week.

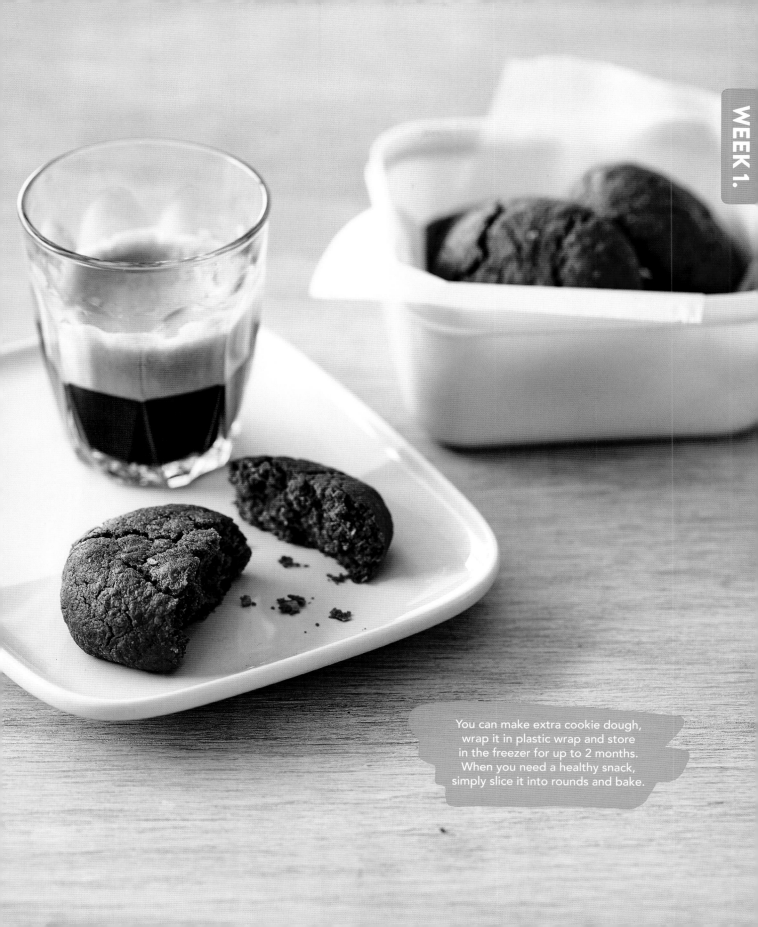

You can make extra cookie dough, wrap it in plastic wrap and store in the freezer for up to 2 months. When you need a healthy snack, simply slice it into rounds and bake.

LEMON AND COCONUT BLISS BALLS

MAKES: 15   **PREPARATION TIME:** 10 MINUTES, PLUS CHILLING TIME

2 ½ cups desiccated coconut
½ cup raw almonds
2 tablespoons honey
80 ml coconut oil, melted
1 tablespoon lemon juice
2 teaspoons finely grated
  lemon zest

NUTRI DETAILS PER SERVE

171 cals/718 kjs
Protein: 1.8 g
Fibre: 2.3 g
Total fat: 16.2 g
Sat fat: 12.5 g
Carbs: 4.2 g
Total sugar: 4.2 g
Free sugar: 3.2 g

Place 2 cups of the desiccated coconut in a food processor, add the almonds, honey, coconut oil, lemon juice and lemon zest and blend for 1 minute. Place the mixture in the fridge for 30 minutes to firm up.

Form the chilled mixture into 15 small balls and roll them in the remaining desiccated coconut. Place on a tray lined with baking paper and chill in the fridge for 30 minutes or until firm. Store in an airtight container in the fridge for a week or freeze for up to a month. One bliss ball is one serve.

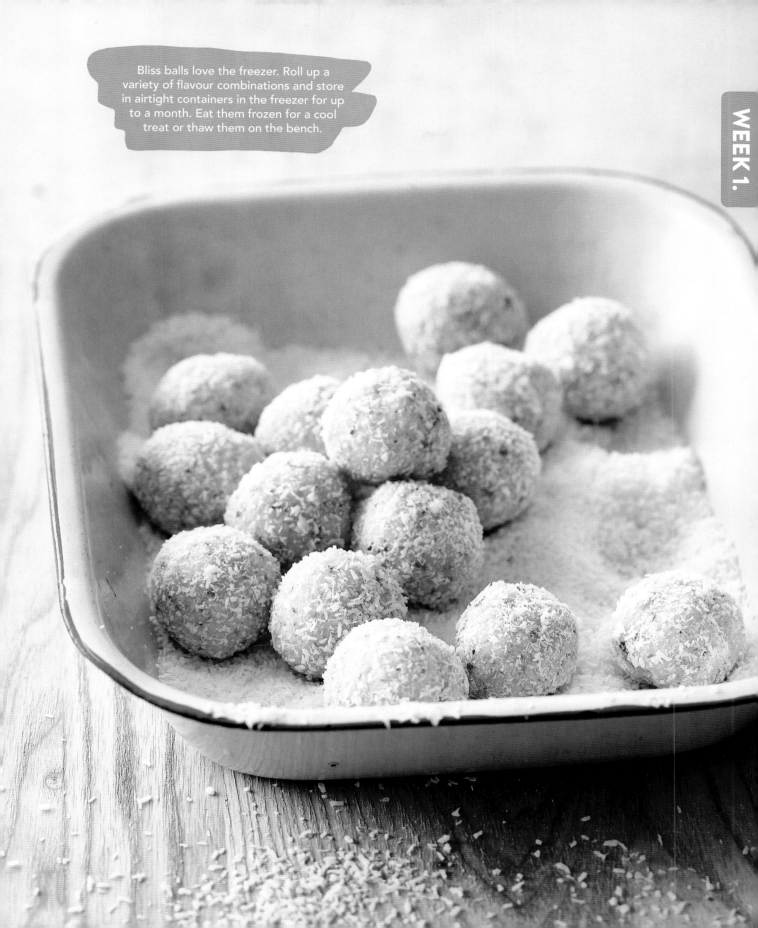

Bliss balls love the freezer. Roll up a variety of flavour combinations and store in airtight containers in the freezer for up to a month. Eat them frozen for a cool treat or thaw them on the bench.

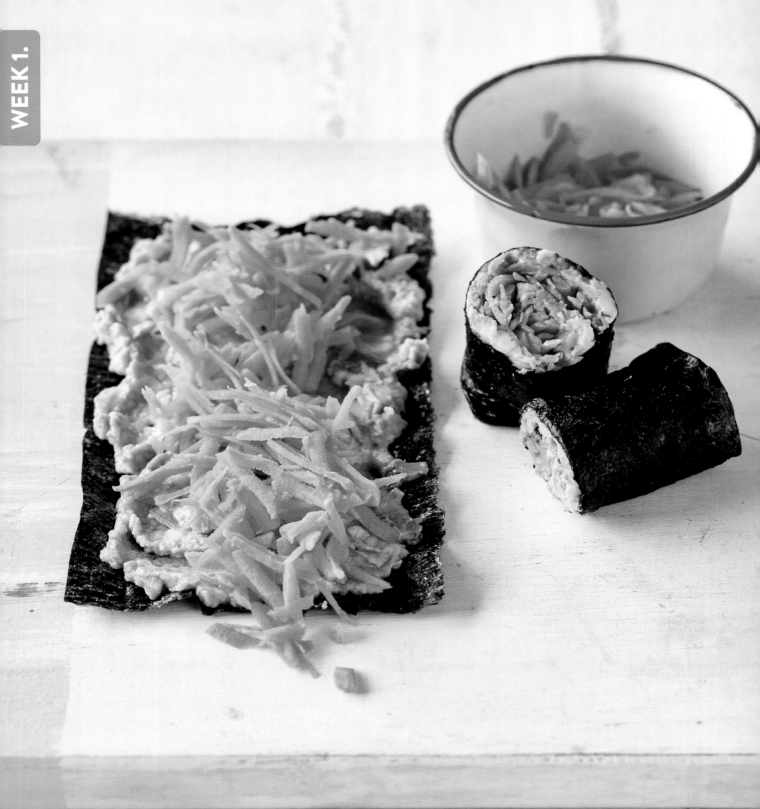

CARROT AND AVOCADO HANDROLLS

SERVES: 1   **PREPARATION TIME:** 5 MINUTES

1 nori sheet
¼ medium avocado, mashed
1 medium carrot, grated

Fold the nori sheet in half to break it into two pieces. Spread the halves with avocado and top with grated carrot.

Roll up like a sushi roll and serve.

NUTRI DETAILS PER SERVE

149 cals/621 kjs
Protein: 2 g
Fibre: 3 g
Total fat: 13 g
Sat fat: 3 g
Carbs: 4 g
Total sugar: 3 g
Free sugar: 0.0 g

STRAWBERRY CHEESECAKE ICE BLOCKS

SERVES: 6   PREPARATION TIME: 10 MINUTES, PLUS FREEZING TIME   COOKING TIME: 1 MINUTE

180 g frozen strawberries

110 g light cream cheese

1 cup reduced-fat Greek-style yoghurt

1 teaspoon vanilla extract

35 g honey

2 teaspoons coconut oil, melted

3 tablespoons rolled oats

1 tablespoon desiccated coconut

NUTRI DETAILS PER SERVE

149 cals/624 kjs
Protein: 5.5 g
Fibre: 2.1 g
Total fat: 8.6 g
Sat fat: 6 g
Carbs: 11.1 g
Total sugar: 9.2 g
Free sugar: 4 g

Place the strawberries in a microwave-safe bowl and microwave for 1 minute or until the berries begin to break down. Transfer to a food processor and process until smooth. Remove one-third of the strawberry mixture from the processor and set aside.

Add the cream cheese, yoghurt, vanilla and 1 tablespoon of the honey to the remaining strawberry mixture in the processor and blend until smooth.

Pour the reserved strawberry mixture evenly into six ice-block moulds, freeze for 1 hour, then pour in the cream cheese mixture.

In a separate bowl, melt the coconut oil and remaining honey in the microwave. Add the oats and desiccated coconut and mix together.

Spoon the oat crumb over each ice block and press gently to smooth it out. Insert an ice-block stick into each mould, then freeze for 6 hours or until firm.

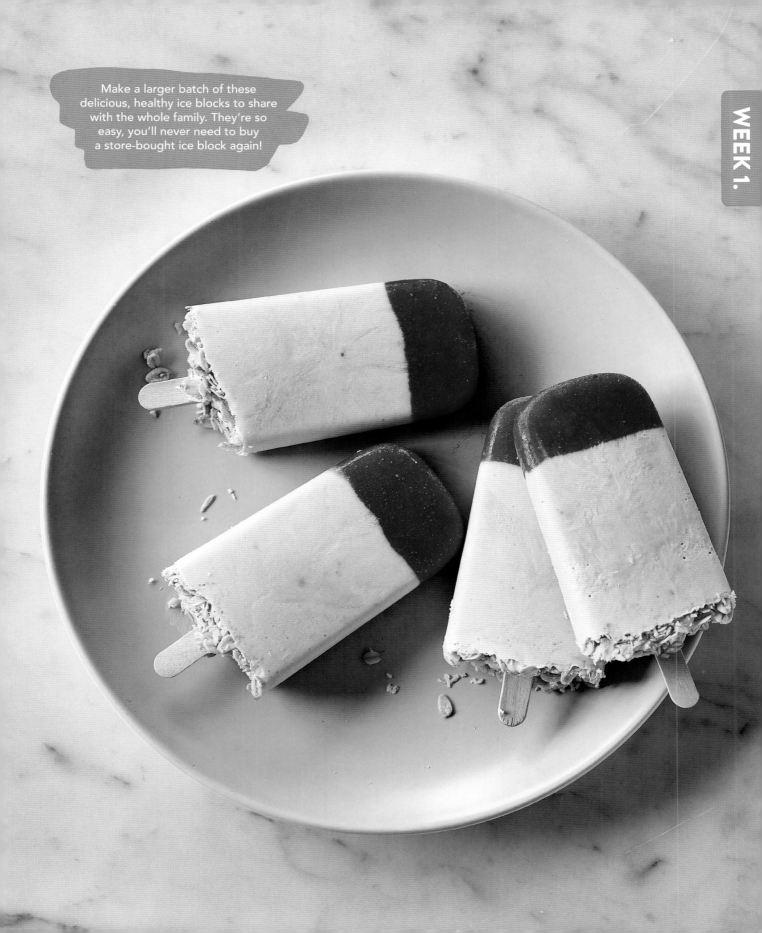

WEEK 1.

Make a larger batch of these delicious, healthy ice blocks to share with the whole family. They're so easy, you'll never need to buy a store-bought ice block again!

WEEK 2.

MEAL & EXERCISE PLAN

2.

	MONDAY	TUESDAY	WEDNESDAY
BREAKFAST	Breakfast Hummingbird Muffins **p.88** 223 cals	Strawberry Cream Oats **p.91** 347 cals	Bacon and Egg Pita Pockets **p.92** 343 cals
MORNING SNACK	Chilli Tuna Dip **p.131** 160 cals	Sweet Potato and Chamomile Crackers **p.132** 178 cals	1 x orange served with 1 cup of herbal tea 54 cals
LUNCH	Rainbow Chopped Salad **p.102** 347 cals	Simple Zucchini and Bacon Slice **p.104** 325 cals	Tropical Brown Rice Salad in a Jar **p.107** 358 cals
EXERCISE	16 minute Tummy Tamer*, Workout 2 (see page 281)	20 minute Body Strong Pilates, Workout 2 (see page 288)	20 minute Deep Core Conditioning*, Workout 2 (see page 291)
AFTERNOON SNACK	Chocolate Muesli Bars **p.134** 197 cals	1 x orange served with 1 cup of herbal tea 54 cals	½ cup Greek-style yoghurt with ½ cup mixed berries 147 cals
DINNER	Fish and Vegetable Curry **p.116** 351 cals	Warm Chicken and Lentil Risoni Salad **p.118** 352 cals	Beef, Ginger and Miso Stir-fry **p.120** 347 cals
EVENING SNACK	½ cup Greek-style yoghurt with ½ cup mixed berries 147 cals	Choc Mint Creams **p.137** 171 cals	Chocolate Muesli Bars **p.134** 197 cals
TOTAL CALORIES	**1425 cals**	**1427 cals**	**1446 cals**

THURSDAY	FRIDAY	SATURDAY	SUNDAY
Herbed Mushrooms and Spinach on Toast **p.94** 365 cals	Matcha Chia Pudding **p.96** 347 cals	Spinach and Feta Puffs **p.99** 309 cals	Baked Mexican Eggs **p.100** 338 cals
Chilli Tuna Dip **p.131** 160 cals	Chilli Tuna Dip **p.131** 160 cals	1 x orange served with 1 cup of herbal tea 54 cals	Sweet Potato and Chamomile Crackers **p.132** 178 cals
Nicoise Salad Open Sandwich **p.108** 440 cals	Chargrilled Pumpkin, Red Onion and Spinach Salad **p.110** 326 cals	Avocado, Green Bean and Salmon Wrap **p.112** 319 cals	Lasagne Soup **p.115** 324 cals
Low Impact 12 minute Total Body Tabata Workout (see page 294)	**20 minute Butt and Thigh*, Workout 2 (see page 299)**	**20 minute Fat Blaster, Workout 2 (see page 303)**	**Active Recovery Day 2 (see page 305)**
Choc-Mint Creams **p.137** 171 cals	1 x orange served with 1 cup of herbal tea 54 cals	Sweet Potato and Chamomile Crackers **p.132** 178 cals	Cheesy Broccoli Bites **p.138** 154 cals
Hidden Veggie Chicken Nuggets and Chips **p.123** 269 cals	Beef Rissoles with Veggies **p.124** 400 cals	One-pot Spaghetti Bolognese **p.126** 415 cals	Slow-cooked Tofu San Choy Bow **p.128** 331 cals
1 orange served with 1 cup of herbal tea 54 cals	½ cup Greek-style yoghurt with ½ cup mixed berries 147 cals	Chocolate Muesli Bars **p.134** 197 cals	Choc Mint Creams **p.137** 171 cals
1459 cals	**1434 cals**	**1472 cals**	**1496 cals**

*Choose the low-impact variation of this workout if you are still recovering from a C-section, abdominal separation, prolapse, or if you have a weak pelvic floor.

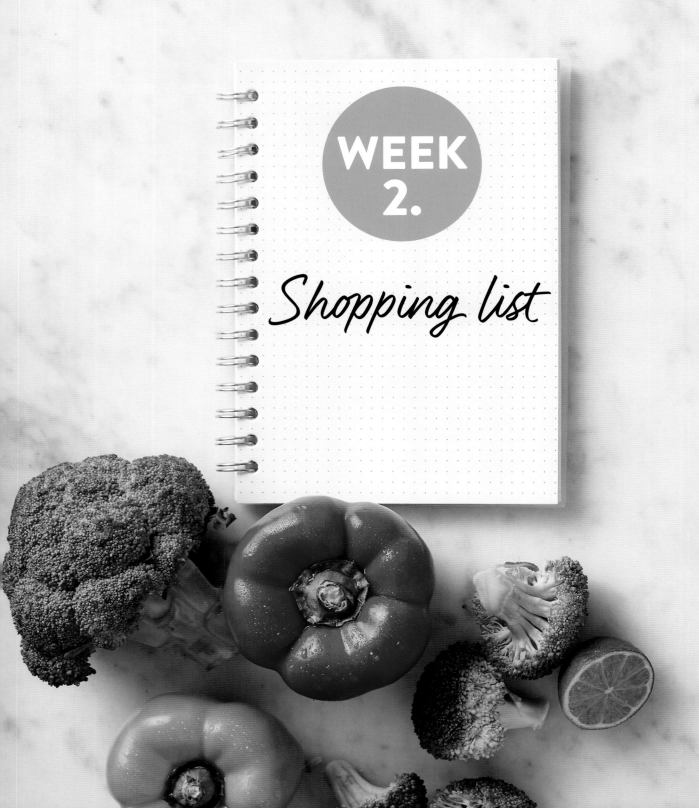

WEEK
2.

Shopping list

Vegetables

Baby spinach leaves 230 g
Beans, green 360 g
Broccoli 800 g
Cabbage, purple 50 g
Capsicums, red 4
Carrots 15
Cauliflower 400 g
Celery 1 bunch
Chilli, bird's eye 1
Corn kernels 500 g (or use tinned)
Cucumber, Lebanese 2
Garlic 16 cloves
Ginger 1 medium knob
Kale 15 g
Lettuce, cos 60 g
Lettuce, iceberg 90 g
Lettuce leaves, mixed 210 g
Mushrooms, small 225 g
Onions, brown 2
Onions, red 2
Pumpkin 450 g
Rocket leaves 120 g
Spring onions 4
Sweet potatoes, small 6
Tomatoes 5
Zucchini 6

Fruit

Apple, red 1
Avocados 2
Bananas 2, 1 frozen
Lemons 2
Lime 1
Medjool dates 140 g
Oranges 5
Pineapple 1
Strawberries 6

Fresh herbs

Basil ½ bunch
Coriander 2 bunches
Flat-leaf parsley 2 bunches
Mint 3 sprigs
Thyme 2 sprigs

Meat, fish and poultry

Bacon rashers, lean and trimmed (4) 110 g
Beef mince, lean 920 g
Beef steak, lean 560 g
Chicken breast fillets 400 g
Chicken mince, lean 400 g
Eggs, free range 21
Fish fillets, white 600 g
Ham, lean, smoked 120 g

Dairy and soy

Cheddar, reduced-fat, grated 70 g
Feta, reduced-fat 80 g
Parmesan, shaved 45 g
Ricotta, reduced-fat 30 g
Tofu, firm 400 g
Yoghurt, reduced-fat natural
  Greek-style 245 g

Breads and grains

Bread of choice, wholemeal
  or gluten free, 6 slices
Mountain bread wraps, wholemeal 2
Pita bread, small wholemeal 2

BREAKFAST HUMMINGBIRD MUFFINS

MAKES 12   PREPARATION TIME: 15 MINUTES   COOKING TIME: 25 MINUTES

100 g fresh pineapple, peeled and cut into small chunks

1 small ripe frozen banana, peeled and roughly chopped

40 g dates, soaked in boiling water for 10 minutes

1 teaspoon vanilla extract

70 g reduced-fat Greek-style yoghurt

1 free-range egg, lightly beaten

2 teaspoons baking powder

½ cup plain wholemeal flour

1 ½ cups LSA (linseed, sunflower and almond meal)

½ cup desiccated coconut

1 teaspoon ground cinnamon

¾ cup walnuts

3 tablespoons honey, to serve

NUTRI DETAILS PER SERVE

223 cals/933 kjs
Protein: 6.5 g
Fibre: 5.8 g
Total fat: 15.3 g
Sat fat: 3.2 g
Carbs: 12.3 g
Total sugar: 8 g
Free sugar: 5 g

Preheat the oven to 180°C. Line a 12-hole standard muffin tin with baking paper or patty pan cases.

In a food processor, blend the pineapple chunks and frozen banana until smooth. Transfer to a large mixing bowl and set aside.

Drain the dates, then transfer to the food processor and process until finely chopped. Add to the mixing bowl, along with the vanilla extract and Greek yoghurt and gently stir to combine. Incorporate the beaten egg.

Sift the baking powder and flour into a separate bowl. Add the LSA, desiccated coconut and cinnamon and stir to combine.

Slowly add the dry ingredients to the wet mixture and gently stir through. Do not overmix or the muffins will be tough.

Spoon the batter evenly among the prepared muffin holes until they're about three-quarters full. Top each muffin with a sprinkle of walnuts.

Bake for 10 minutes or until the tops are browned, then remove from the oven and cover with foil. Return to the oven and bake for a further 10–15 minutes, or until a skewer inserted into a muffin comes out clean. Avoid opening the oven during baking or the muffins will sink.

Allow to cool in the tin for 5 minutes, then turn out onto a wire rack to cool completely.

Serve with a little honey drizzled over the top of each muffin.

One muffin is one serve. Store the muffins in an airtight container in the fridge for up to 4 days or in the freezer for up to 2 months.

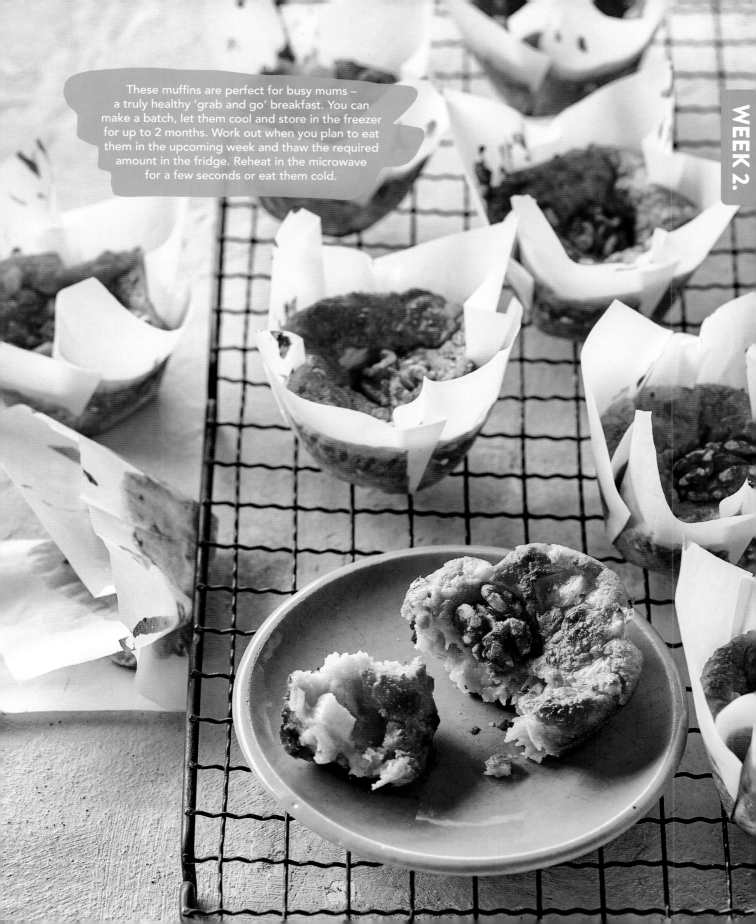

These muffins are perfect for busy mums – a truly healthy 'grab and go' breakfast. You can make a batch, let them cool and store in the freezer for up to 2 months. Work out when you plan to eat them in the upcoming week and thaw the required amount in the fridge. Reheat in the microwave for a few seconds or eat them cold.

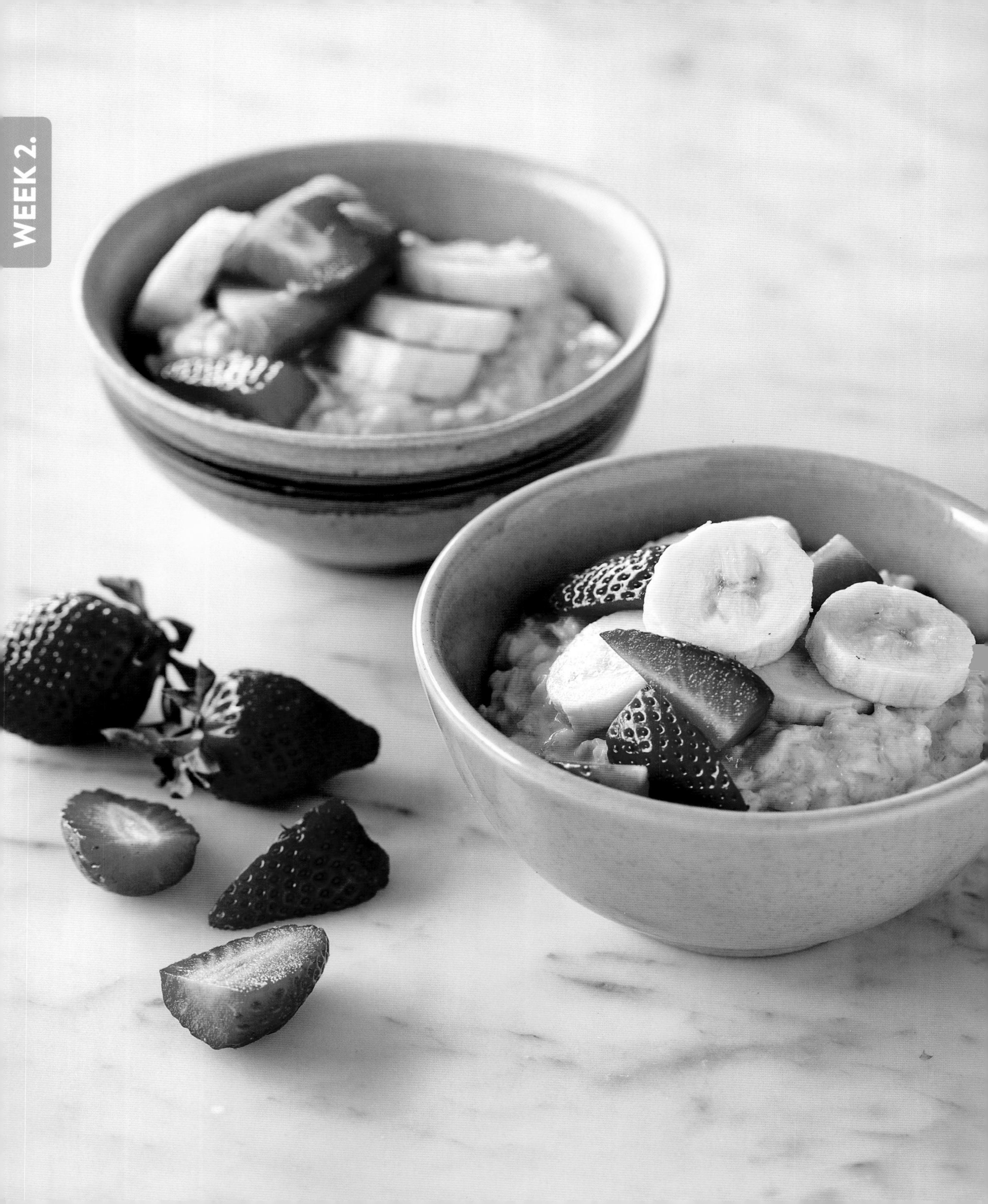

STRAWBERRY CREAM OATS

SERVES: 2   **PREPARATION TIME:** 5 MINUTES   **COOKING TIME:** 5 MINUTES

---

1 cup rolled oats

2 cups reduced-fat milk of choice

2 teaspoons vanilla extract

6 strawberries, sliced

1 small banana, sliced

Combine the oats and milk in a saucepan and cook, stirring, over medium–low heat for 3–5 minutes or until thick and creamy.

When the oats are ready, stir in the vanilla and pour into two bowls. Top with the sliced strawberry and banana and serve.

NUTRI DETAILS PER SERVE

347 cals/1459 kjs
Protein: 16 g
Fibre: 4.6 g
Total fat: 7.7 g
Sat fat: 3 g
Carbs: 51.6 g
Total sugar: 21 g
Free sugar: 0.0 g

BACON AND EGG PITA POCKETS

SERVES: 2   **PREPARATION TIME:** 5 MINUTES   **COOKING TIME:** 10 MINUTES

2 free-range eggs
2 teaspoons reduced-fat milk
   of choice
cooking oil spray
2 lean bacon rashers, trimmed
2 small wholemeal pita breads
20 g baby spinach leaves

NUTRI DETAILS PER SERVE

343 cals/1444 kjs
Protein: 18.6 g
Fibre: 4.7 g
Total fat: 13.9 g
Sat fat: 5.8 g
Carbs: 33.8 g
Total sugar: 2.6 g
Free sugar: 0.0 g

Beat together the eggs and milk in a bowl.

Spray a medium frying pan with cooking oil spray and place over medium–high heat. Add the egg mixture and gently scrape across the pan with a flat spatula until the egg is cooked and scrambled. Remove from the pan and set aside.

Add the bacon and cook for 2–3 minutes each side or until cooked and crisp.

Slice open the pita breads and fill with the spinach, scrambled egg and bacon to serve.

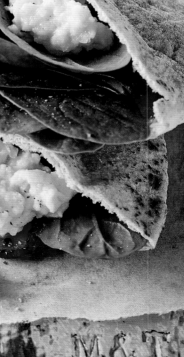

HERBED MUSHROOMS AND SPINACH ON TOAST

SERVES: 2   **PREPARATION TIME:** 10 MINUTES   **COOKING TIME:** 10 MINUTES

1 tablespoon extra-virgin olive oil

2 teaspoons fresh thyme leaves

1 garlic clove, finely chopped

150 g mushrooms, sliced

salt and freshly ground black pepper

60 g baby spinach leaves

2 slices wholegrain or gluten-free bread of choice

½ medium avocado

Heat 3 teaspoons of the olive oil in a medium saucepan over medium heat. Add the thyme and half the garlic clove and cook, stirring, for 2 minutes. Add the mushrooms, season with salt and pepper and cook until nicely browned. Add 2 tablespoons water, then cover and cook for 4–5 minutes or until tender.

Meanwhile, heat the remaining olive oil in a separate saucepan over medium heat. Add the spinach and remaining garlic and give it a good stir. Cover and cook for 3–4 minutes, stirring occasionally, until the spinach has wilted. Season with salt and pepper

Toast the bread and spread with the avocado. Place one piece on each plate, top with the spinach and mushrooms and serve.

NUTRI DETAILS PER SERVE

365 cals/1532 kjs
Protein: 18 g
Fibre: 21 g
Total fat: 21 g
Sat fat: 4 g
Carbs: 20 g
Total sugar: 3 g
Free sugar: 0.0 g

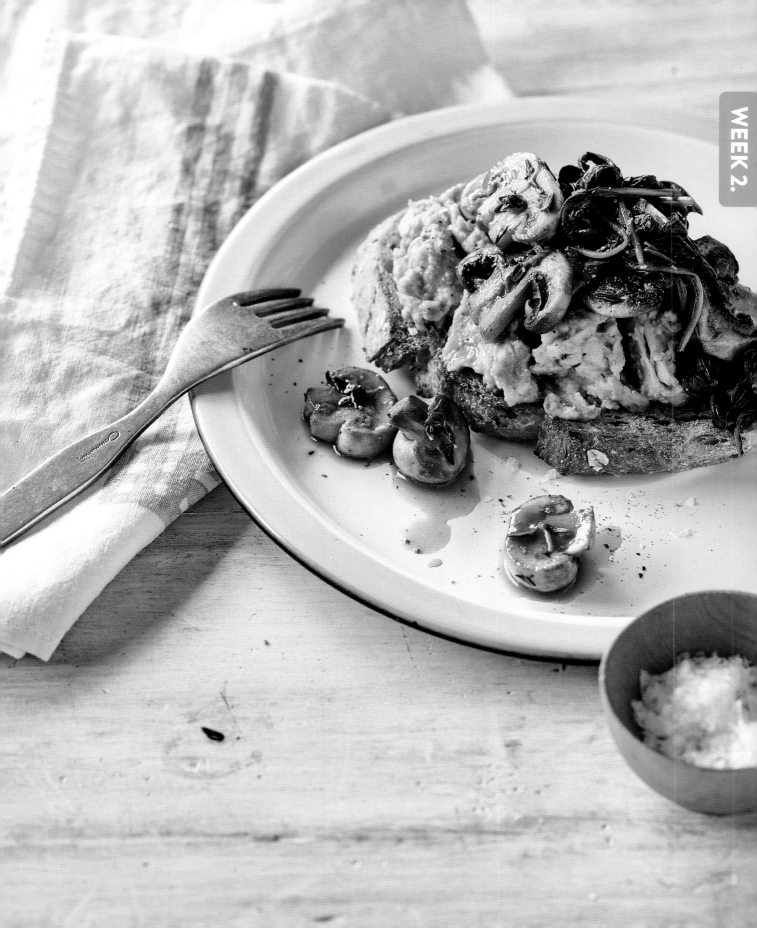

MATCHA CHIA PUDDING

SERVES: 2 **PREPARATION TIME:** 5 MINUTES, PLUS CHILLING TIME

⅓ cup chia seeds, plus extra
   to sprinkle
2 cups reduced-fat milk of
   choice
2 tablespoons rolled oats
2 tablespoons pure maple syrup
2 teaspoons vanilla extract
1 teaspoon matcha green tea
   powder

Place half the chia seeds in a food processor. Add the milk, oats, maple syrup, vanilla and matcha powder and blitz until smooth.

Spoon the mixture into two serving glasses or bowls and stir in the remaining chia seeds. Cover and refrigerate overnight until thick and creamy. Sprinkle with extra chia seeds before serving.

NUTRI DETAILS PER SERVE

347 cals/1453 kjs
Protein: 16.5 g
Fibre: 11.7 g
Total fat: 14 g
Sat fat: 3.5 g
Carbs: 33.5 g
Total sugar: 23.2 g
Free sugar: 8.9 g

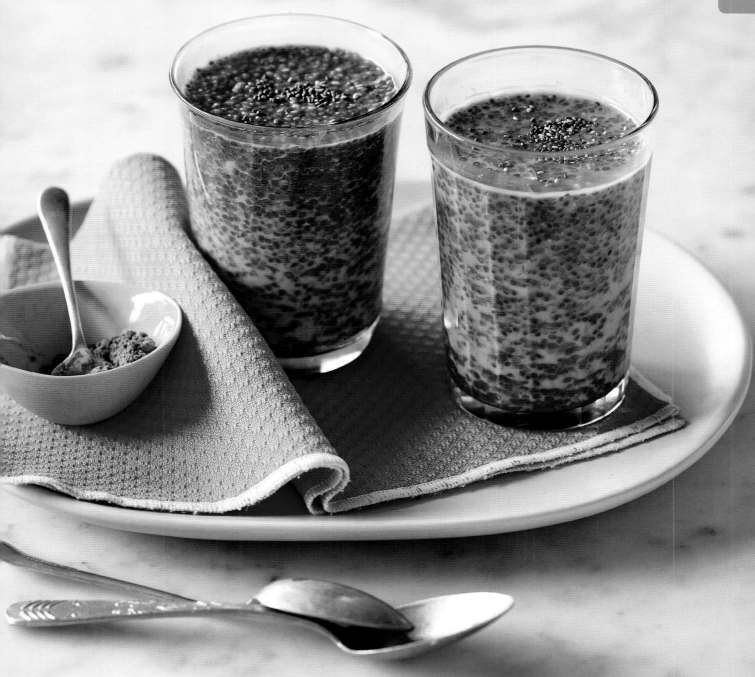

Make a larger batch of these puddings and store them in the fridge for 3–4 days. You will have a healthy, delicious breakfast ready in seconds every morning.

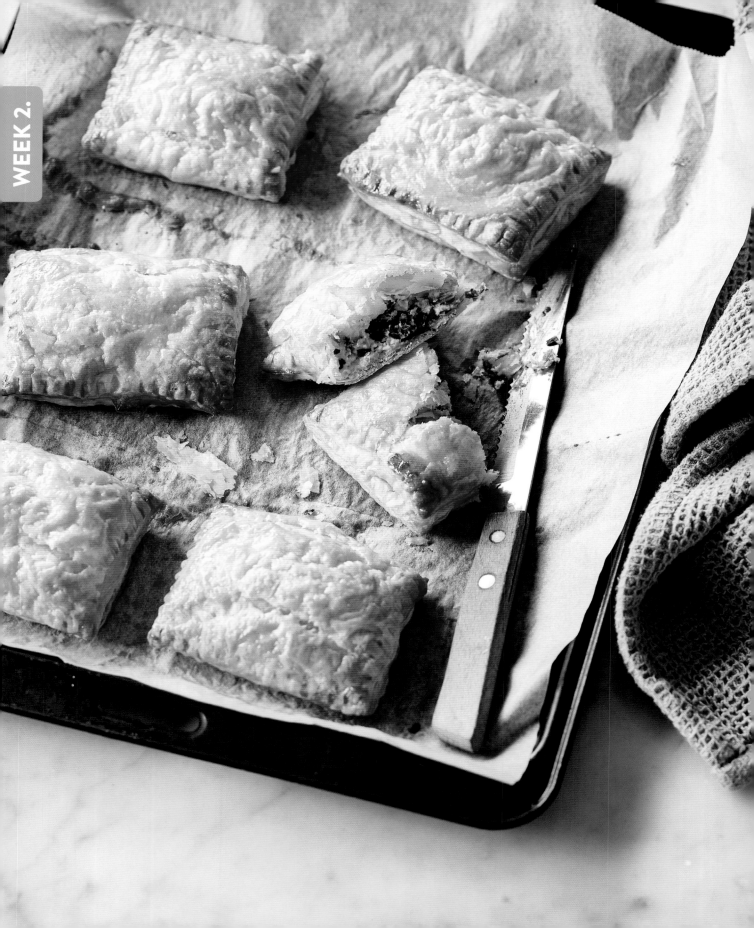

SPINACH AND FETA PUFFS

SERVES: 3   **PREPARATION TIME:** 15 MINUTES   **COOKING TIME:** 25 MINUTES

60 g frozen spinach, thawed
80 g reduced-fat feta
1 garlic clove, minced
2 free-range eggs
freshly ground black pepper
1 sheet reduced-fat puff pastry

NUTRI DETAILS PER SERVE

309 cals/1296 kjs
Protein: 15.7 g
Fibre: 2.5 g
Total fat: 17.1 g
Sat fat: 9.1 g
Carbs: 22.2 g
Total sugar: 1.4 g
Free sugar: 0.0 g

Preheat the oven to 200°C and line a baking tray with baking paper.

Squeeze the excess water from the thawed spinach, then place in a bowl with the feta, garlic and one of the eggs. Mix well and season with pepper.

Cut the just-thawed pastry into six rectangles. Place a spoonful of spinach filling on one half of a rectangle, fold the other half over the filling and crimp the pastry edges with a fork to seal. Repeat with the remaining pastry rectangles and filling.

Place the puffs on the prepared tray. Whisk the remaining egg in a small bowl and brush over each pastry. Bake for 25 minutes or until golden and cooked through.

One serve is two puffs. The pastries can be made ahead of time and stored in the fridge to reheat later, or may be frozen. Just thaw and reheat in the oven to serve.

BAKED MEXICAN EGGS

SERVES: 2   **PREPARATION TIME:** 10 MINUTES   **COOKING TIME:** 20 MINUTES

cooking oil spray

200 g tinned tomatoes

200 g tinned kidney beans, drained and rinsed

1 teaspoon salt-reduced taco seasoning

4 free-range eggs

⅓ cup grated reduced-fat cheddar

2 tablespoons coriander leaves

Preheat the oven to 180°C. Lightly spray two individual ovenproof dishes with cooking oil spray (or use a larger dish to fit the number of serves you are preparing).

Mix together the tomatoes, beans and taco seasoning and place in the prepared dishes. Make two indents in each serve with the back of a spoon, then crack an egg into each indent and sprinkle with grated cheese.

Bake for 15–20 minutes or until the eggs are cooked through. Sprinkle with coriander and serve.

NUTRI DETAILS PER SERVE

338 cals/1418 kjs

Protein: 31 g

Fibre: 9 g

Total fat: 13 g

Sat fat: 4.5 g

Carbs: 21 g

Total sugar: 8.7 g

Free sugar: 0.0 g

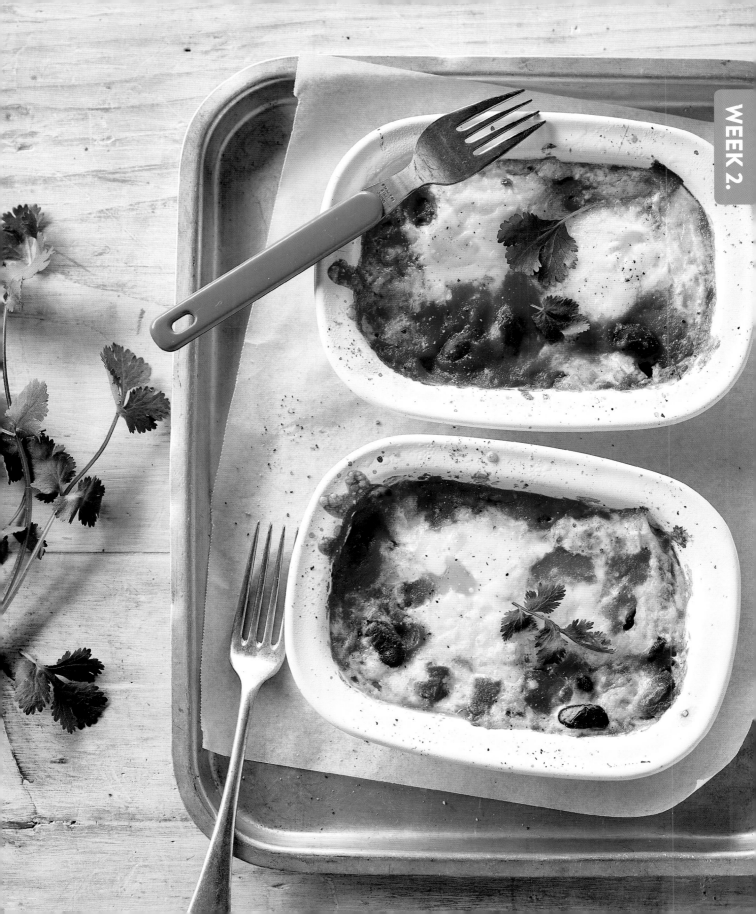

RAINBOW CHOPPED SALAD

SERVES: 2   **PREPARATION TIME:** 10 MINUTES, PLUS MARINATING TIME

200 g cauliflower, cut into florets

60 g mixed lettuce leaves, chopped

50 g shredded purple cabbage

½ cup chopped flat-leaf parsley leaves

3 tablespoons chopped coriander leaves

1 small apple, cored and chopped

⅓ cup walnuts, chopped

½ medium avocado, diced

1 tablespoon lemon juice

1 tablespoon extra virgin olive oil

Place all the ingredients in a large bowl and toss together well. Set aside to marinate for at least 15 minutes.

Divide between two plates and serve.

NUTRI DETAILS PER SERVE

347 cals/1453 kjs
Protein: 7 g
Fibre: 8.2 g
Total fat: 29.8 g
Sat fat: 3.7 g
Carbs: 9 g
Total sugar: 8.9 g
Free sugar: 0.0 g

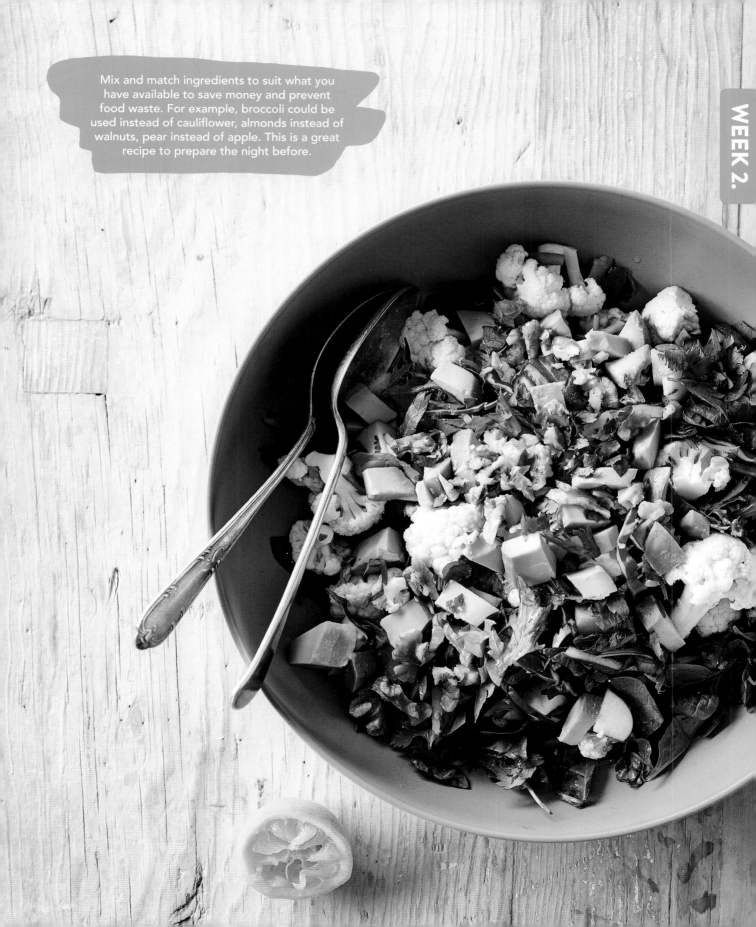

Mix and match ingredients to suit what you have available to save money and prevent food waste. For example, broccoli could be used instead of cauliflower, almonds instead of walnuts, pear instead of apple. This is a great recipe to prepare the night before.

SIMPLE ZUCCHINI AND BACON SLICE

SERVES: 2   **PREPARATION TIME:** 10 MINUTES   **COOKING TIME:** 30 MINUTES

cooking oil spray

2 lean bacon rashers, trimmed and diced

1 small zucchini, grated

1 medium carrot, grated

⅓ cup chopped flat-leaf parsley leaves

4 free-range eggs, lightly beaten

2 tablespoons plain wholemeal flour

2 tablespoons grated reduced-fat cheddar

freshly ground black pepper

Preheat the oven to 170°C and lightly spray a small slice tin with cooking oil spray.

Combine the bacon, grated vegetables, parsley, egg, flour and grated cheese to form a batter. Season well with pepper.

Pour the batter into the prepared dish and bake for 25–30 minutes until golden and set in the centre. Allow to cool slightly before cutting into slices to serve.

NUTRI DETAILS PER SERVE

325 cals/1361 kjs
Protein: 27 g
Fibre: 4 g
Total fat: 19 g
Sat fat: 7 g
Carbs: 10 g
Total sugar: 3 g
Free sugar: 0.0 g

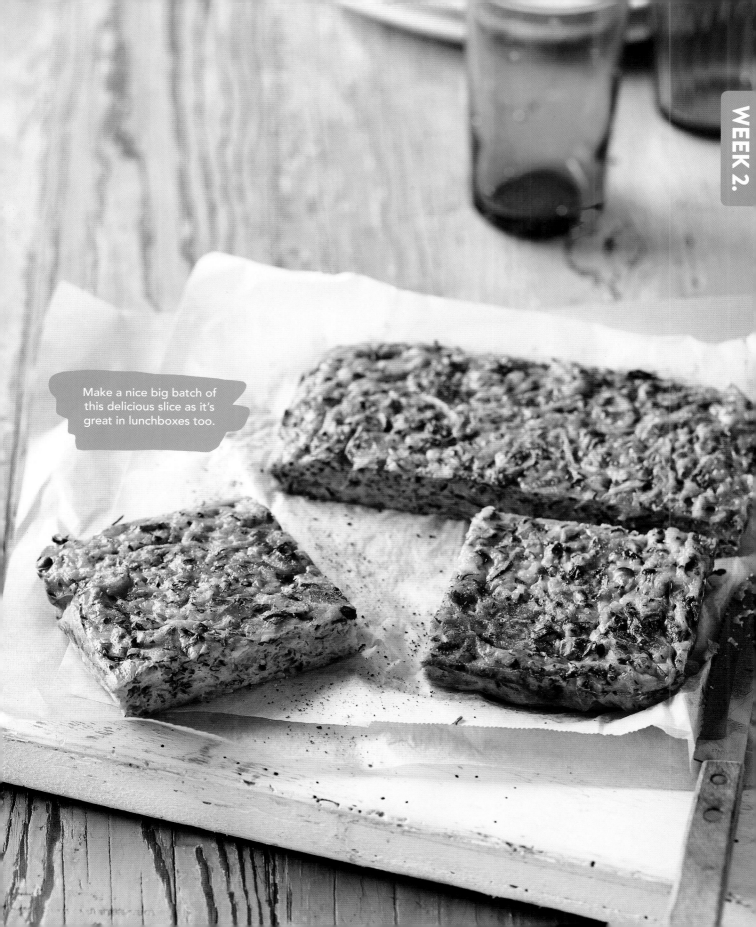

Make a nice big batch of this delicious slice as it's great in lunchboxes too.

If you are using tinned pineapple for this recipe use the juice from the tin for the dressing, rather than purchasing a separate container of pineapple juice, or replace it with lemon juice if you prefer.

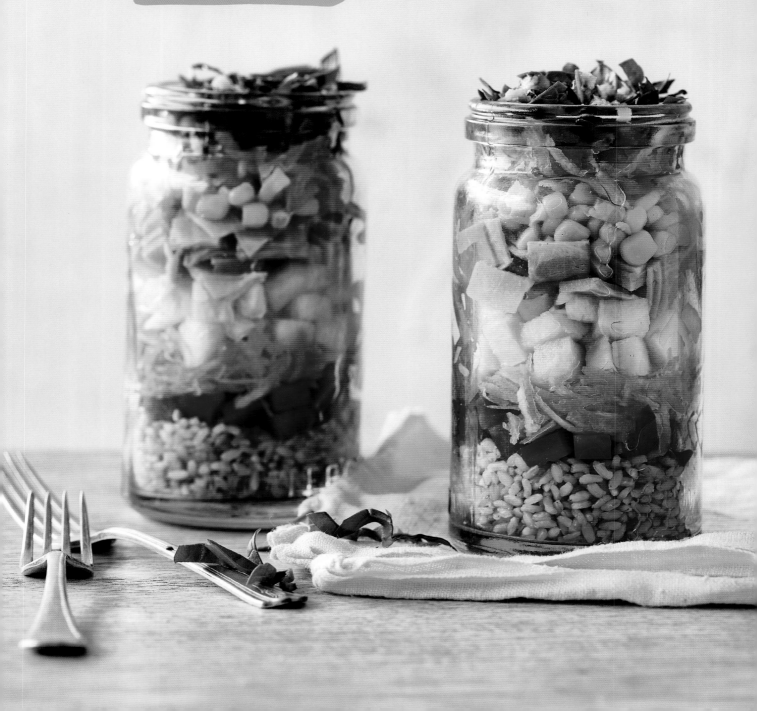

TROPICAL BROWN RICE SALAD IN A JAR

SERVES: 2 **PREPARATION TIME:** 10 MINUTES, PLUS CHILLING TIME **COOKING TIME:** 45 MINUTES

½ cup brown rice

½ red capsicum, seeds removed, diced

1 medium carrot, grated

110 g peeled pineapple (fresh or tinned), diced

6 slices lean smoked ham, chopped

½ cup corn kernels (fresh or tinned)

30 g baby spinach, chopped

1 tablespoon unsweetened pineapple juice

1 garlic clove, crushed

½ teaspoon grated ginger

½ teaspoon extra virgin olive oil

Bring 2 cups water to the boil in a medium saucepan, add the rice and simmer for 45 minutes or until tender. Drain and set aside to cool.

Spoon the rice evenly into two mason jars (or lunchbox containers with lids). Divide the remaining ingredients between the jars and either leave them in separate layers or shake gently to combine.

If possible, prepare the salad in the morning and let it rest in the fridge for several hours, shaking occasionally, so the flavours combine and develop.

Turn out into bowls and serve.

NUTRI DETAILS PER SERVE

358 cals/1505 kjs
Protein: 18.5 g
Fibre: 5.6 g
Total fat: 5.2 g
Sat fat: 1.3 g
Carbs: 56.2 g
Total sugar: 11.2 g
Free sugar: 1 g

NICOISE SALAD OPEN SANDWICH

SERVES: 2   PREPARATION TIME: 10 MINUTES   COOKING TIME: 15 MINUTES

1 teaspoon Dijon mustard

2 tablespoons reduced-fat Greek-style yoghurt

2 teaspoons extra virgin olive oil

180 g tinned tuna in spring water, drained

4 slices wholegrain or gluten-free bread of choice

60 g cos lettuce leaves, roughly chopped

1 tomato, sliced

60 g green beans, trimmed, roughly chopped

6 kalamata olives, sliced

2 hard-boiled free-range eggs, peeled and sliced

Combine the mustard, yoghurt and olive oil in a small bowl. Stir in the tuna.

Toast the bread and place two slices on each plate. Top with the lettuce, tomato, tuna mixture, beans, olives and egg and serve.

NUTRI DETAILS PER SERVE

440 cals/1848 kjs
Protein: 39 g
Fibre: 7 g
Total fat: 15 g
Sat fat: 4 g
Carbs: 36 g
Total sugar: 7 g
Free sugar: 0.0 g

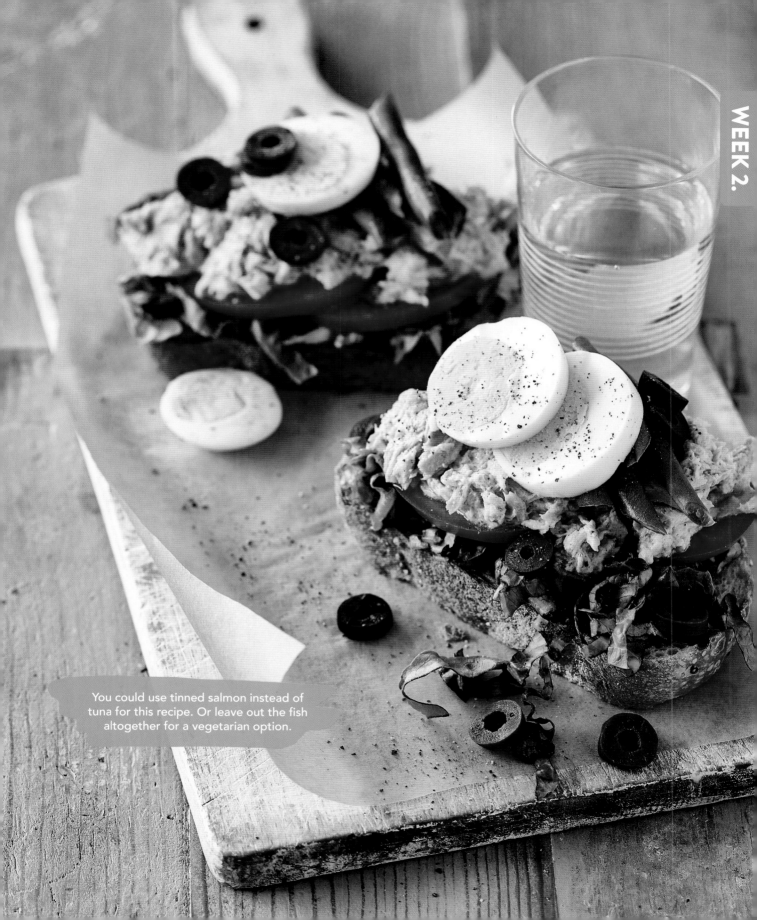

You could use tinned salmon instead of tuna for this recipe. Or leave out the fish altogether for a vegetarian option.

CHARGRILLED PUMPKIN, RED ONION AND SPINACH SALAD

SERVES: 2   **PREPARATION TIME:** 10 MINUTES   **COOKING TIME:** 12 MINUTES

2 tablespoons pumpkin seeds

1 teaspoon ground cumin

1 teaspoon smoked paprika

1 tablespoon lime juice, plus extra if needed

1 tablespoon chopped coriander leaves

2 tablespoons extra virgin olive oil, plus extra if needed

450 g pumpkin, peeled, seeds removed and finely sliced

¼ red onion, sliced into wedges

60 g baby spinach leaves

NUTRI DETAILS PER SERVE

326 cals/1363 kjs

Protein: 8.1 g

Fibre: 5.2 g

Total fat: 27.1 g

Sat fat: 4.2 g

Carbs: 10.6 g

Total sugar: 7.9 g

Free sugar: 0.0 g

Roast the pumpkin seeds in a dry frying pan over low heat, then set aside to cool.

Place the pumpkin seeds, cumin, paprika, lime juice, coriander and half the olive oil in a food processor or blender and process until smooth. Add a little more olive oil, lime juice or water to loosen if needed.

Heat a chargrill pan or frying pan over medium–high heat.

Brush the pumpkin slices with the remaining olive oil, then add to the pan and cook for 1–2 minutes each side or until tender. Transfer to a plate.

Add the onion to the pan and cook for 2 minutes each side or until lightly charred. Set aside to cool slightly.

Arrange the spinach, pumpkin and onion on two serving plates. Drizzle with the pumpkin seed dressing and serve.

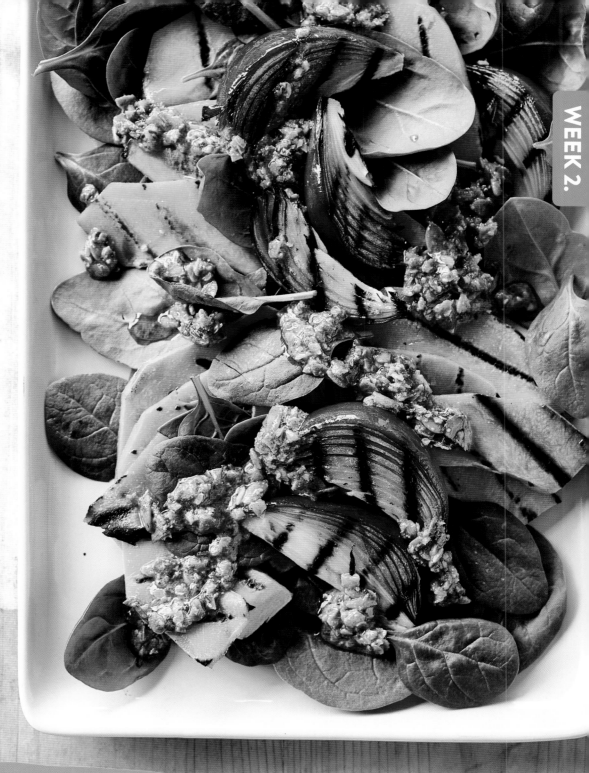

Prepare a larger batch of the pumpkin seed dressing ahead of time and store it in a jar in the fridge for up to a week. It's great drizzled over cooked chicken breast, tossed through wholemeal pasta with some veggies, or even dolloped on a homemade pizza.

AVOCADO, GREEN BEAN AND SALMON WRAP

SERVES: 2   **PREPARATION TIME:** 10 MINUTES

½ medium avocado, mashed

100 g tinned salmon in spring water, drained

2 teaspoons lemon juice

2 wholemeal mountain bread wraps

60 g green beans, trimmed and halved lengthways

½ medium carrot, grated

30 g mixed lettuce leaves

Combine the avocado, salmon and lemon juice in a small bowl.

Spread the salmon mixture onto the mountain bread wraps and top with the beans, grated carrot and lettuce leaves. Roll up to enclose the filling and serve.

NUTRI DETAILS PER SERVE

319 cals/1339 kjs
Protein: 9.5 g
Fibre: 5 g
Total fat: 11 g
Sat fat: 2.3 g
Carbs: 36.4 g
Total sugar: 3.1 g
Free sugar: 0.0 g

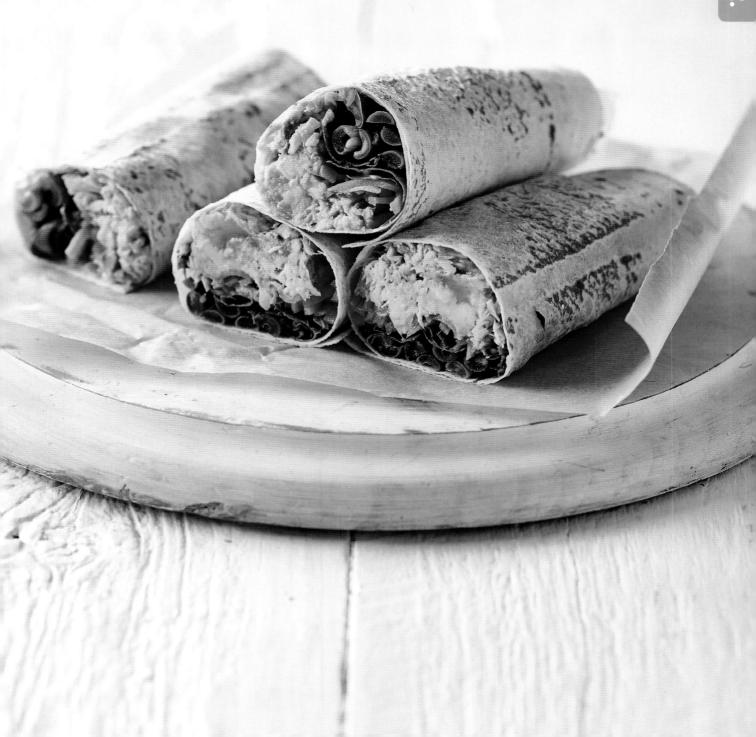

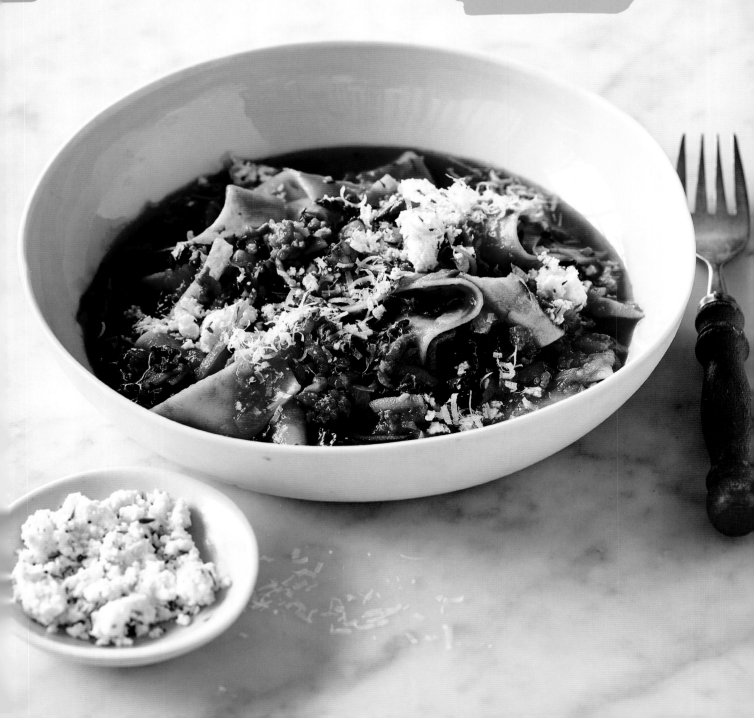

This recipe would also work well with lean pork or chicken mince if you prefer.

LASAGNE SOUP

SERVES: 2   **PREPARATION TIME:** 10 MINUTES   **COOKING TIME:** 35 MINUTES

2 teaspoons extra virgin olive oil

100 g lean beef mince

½ brown onion, diced

1 garlic clove, sliced

15 g kale leaves, finely chopped

1 medium carrot, grated

1 small zucchini, grated

1 cup tomato passata

2 cups salt-reduced beef stock

2 dried lasagne sheets

2 tablespoons reduced-fat ricotta

1 teaspoon finely grated lemon zest

¼ teaspoon dried thyme

1 teaspoon grated parmesan

NUTRI DETAILS PER SERVE

324 cals/1359 kjs
Protein: 23 g
Fibre: 6.5 g
Total fat: 12.5 g
Sat fat: 6.5 g
Carbs: 26 g
Total sugar: 10 g
Free sugar: 0.0 g

Heat the olive oil in a medium saucepan over medium–high heat, add the mince and onion and cook for 1–2 minutes or until the mince is nicely browned, breaking up any lumps with the back of a wooden spoon. Add the garlic, kale, carrot and zucchini and stir to combine, then cook for 2 minutes or until the vegetables start to soften.

Add the tomato passata and stock. Bring to the boil, then reduce the heat and simmer for 10 minutes. Break up the lasagne sheets, add to the pan and simmer for a further 20 minutes.

Meanwhile, mix together the ricotta, lemon zest and thyme in a small bowl.

Pour the soup into two bowls, top with the ricotta mixture and grated parmesan and serve.

VARIATION, USING A SLOW-COOKER: Heat the olive oil in a medium saucepan over medium–high heat, add the mince and onion and cook for 1–2 minutes or until the mince is nicely browned, breaking up any lumps with the back of a wooden spoon. Transfer the mince mixture to the slow-cooker. Add the garlic, kale, carrot, zucchini, passata and stock and cook on low for 8 hours, adding the broken lasagne sheets in the final 40 minutes of cooking. Mix together the ricotta, lemon zest and thyme in a small bowl. To serve, pour the soup into bowls and top with the ricotta mixture and grated parmesan.

FISH AND VEGETABLE CURRY

SERVES: 4   PREPARATION TIME: 10 MINUTES   COOKING TIME: 10 MINUTES

2 tablespoons coconut oil

4 garlic cloves, minced

1 tablespoon grated ginger

2 tablespoons red curry paste

1 cup reduced-fat coconut milk

2 red capsicums, seeds removed, sliced

200 g broccoli, cut into florets

600 g white fish fillet of choice, skin and bones removed, cut into 3 cm cubes

⅓ cup coriander leaves

Melt the coconut oil in a medium saucepan over medium–high heat, add the garlic and cook for 1 minute. Add the ginger and curry paste and cook for a further 30 seconds or until fragrant. Pour in the coconut milk and 1 cup water and stir to combine.

Add the capsicum, broccoli and fish and simmer for 4–5 minutes or until the fish is cooked through and the vegetables are tender.

Spoon the curry into four bowls and serve sprinkled with coriander.

NUTRI DETAILS PER SERVE

351 cals/1475 kjs
Protein: 35 g
Fibre: 4.1 g
Total fat: 20.5 g
Sat fat: 14 g
Carbs: 5.6 g
Total sugar: 4.1 g
Free sugar: 0.0 g

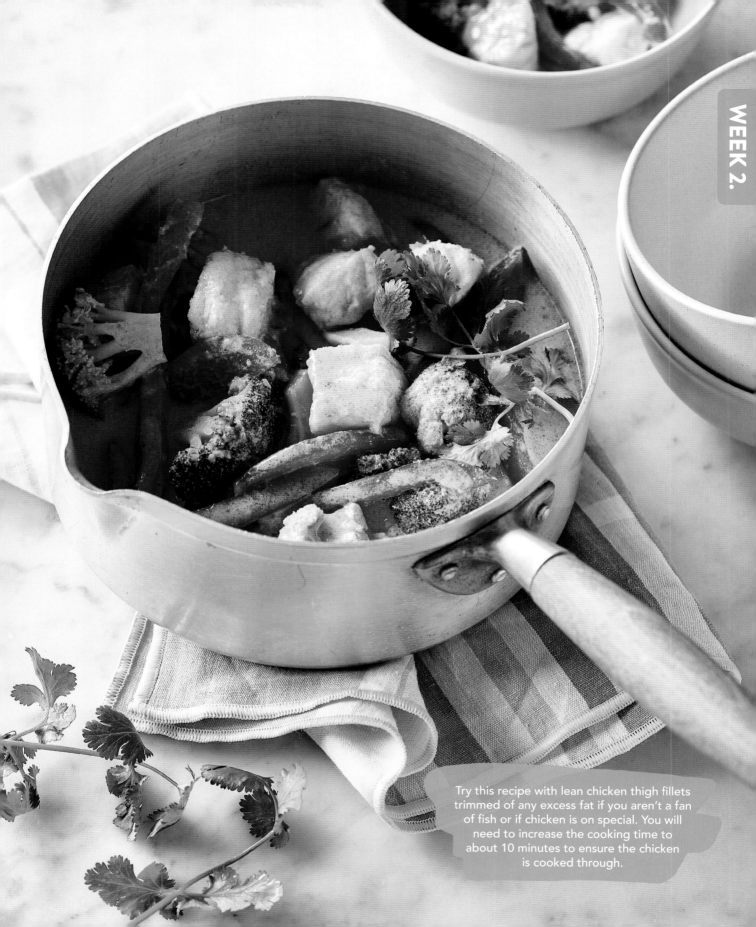

Try this recipe with lean chicken thigh fillets trimmed of any excess fat if you aren't a fan of fish or if chicken is on special. You will need to increase the cooking time to about 10 minutes to ensure the chicken is cooked through.

WARM CHICKEN AND LENTIL RISONI SALAD

SERVES: 4   **PREPARATION TIME:** 15 MINUTES   **COOKING TIME:** 20 MINUTES

2 × 200 g chicken breast fillets
2 garlic cloves, crushed
2 teaspoons extra virgin olive oil
1 teaspoon smoked paprika
1 teaspoon ground cumin
1 teaspoon ground turmeric
⅔ cup risoni
80 g tinned brown lentils, drained and rinsed
2 tomatoes, chopped
⅓ cup flat-leaf parsley leaves
⅓ cup chopped mint leaves
120 g rocket leaves
⅓ cup reduced-fat Greek-style yoghurt
1 tablespoon tahini
1 tablespoon lemon juice

Preheat the oven to 180°C.

In a bowl, coat the chicken in the garlic, olive oil, paprika, cumin and turmeric. Place in a roasting dish and bake for 15–20 minutes or until golden brown and cooked through.

Meanwhile, cook the risoni in a saucepan of boiling water for 8–10 minutes or until al dente. Drain well.

Combine the warm risoni, lentils, tomato, parsley, mint and rocket leaves in a bowl.

Whisk together the yoghurt, tahini and lemon juice.

Divide the risoni mixture among four bowls. Thickly slice the chicken and arrange it on top of the warm salad. Serve drizzled with the yoghurt dressing.

NUTRI DETAILS PER SERVE

352 cals/1472 kjs
Protein: 28.6 g
Fibre: 5.1 g
Total fat: 15.4 g
Sat fat: 3.9 g
Carbs: 21.4 g
Total sugar: 3.3 g
Free sugar: 0.0 g

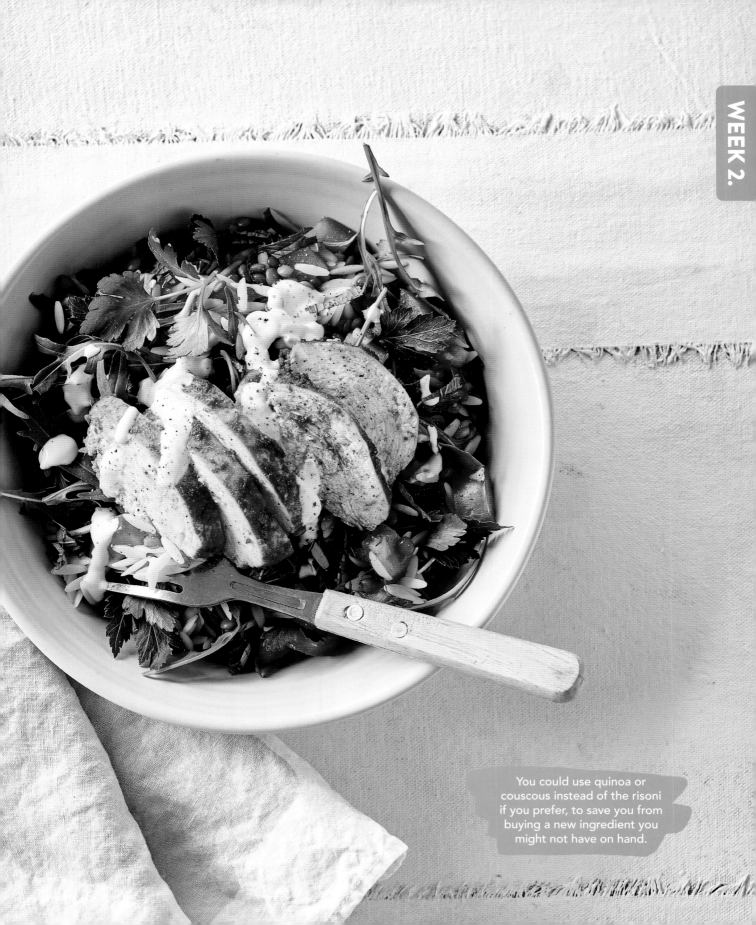

You could use quinoa or couscous instead of the risoni if you prefer, to save you from buying a new ingredient you might not have on hand.

BEEF, GINGER AND MISO STIR-FRY

SERVES: 4   PREPARATION TIME: 10 MINUTES   COOKING TIME: 10 MINUTES

2 tablespoons coconut oil

2 teaspoons grated ginger

½ teaspoon dried chilli flakes

1 tablespoon miso paste
(from the Asian section of
the supermarket)

560 g lean beef steak of choice,
finely sliced

400 g broccoli, cut into florets

4 medium carrots, finely sliced

4 spring onions, finely sliced

⅓ cup coriander leaves

Heat a wok or frying pan over medium heat, add the coconut oil, ginger, chilli and miso paste and stir-fry for about 30 seconds. Add the beef and stir-fry for 3 minutes, then remove from the wok.

Add the broccoli, carrot and half the spring onion to the wok and stir-fry for 3–4 minutes or until the broccoli is bright green and the vegetables are crisp–tender. Return the beef to the wok and toss well to combine.

Divide the stir-fry among four bowls, top with the remaining spring onion and the coriander and serve.

NUTRI DETAILS PER SERVE

347 cals/1456 kjs
Protein: 35 g
Fibre: 6 g
Total fat: 19 g
Sat fat: 14.5 g
Carbs: 5 g
Total sugar: 4 g
Free sugar: 0.0 g

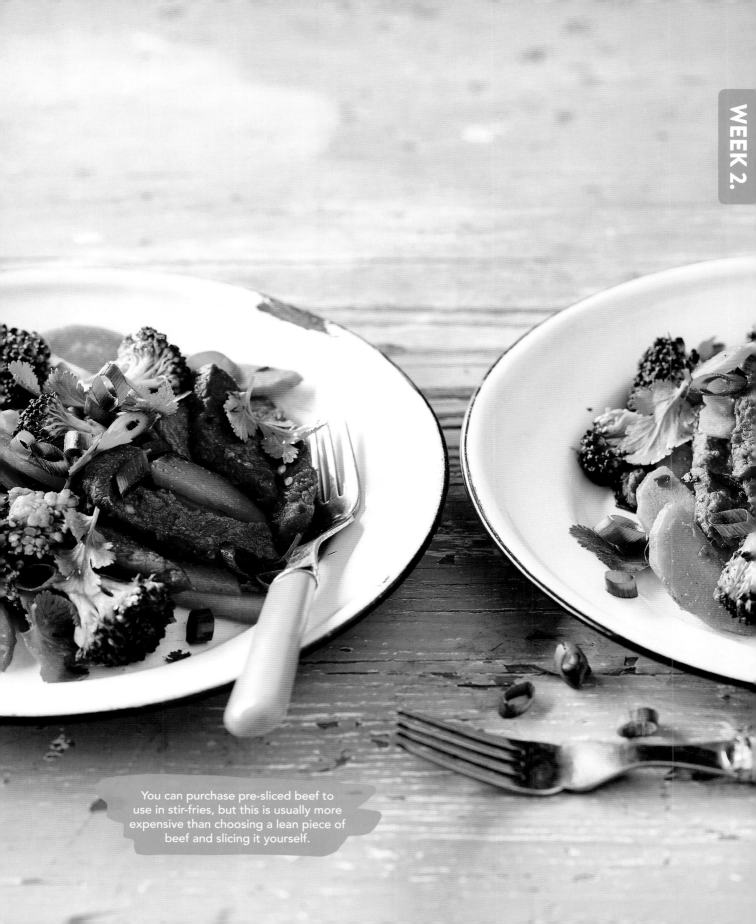

You can purchase pre-sliced beef to use in stir-fries, but this is usually more expensive than choosing a lean piece of beef and slicing it yourself.

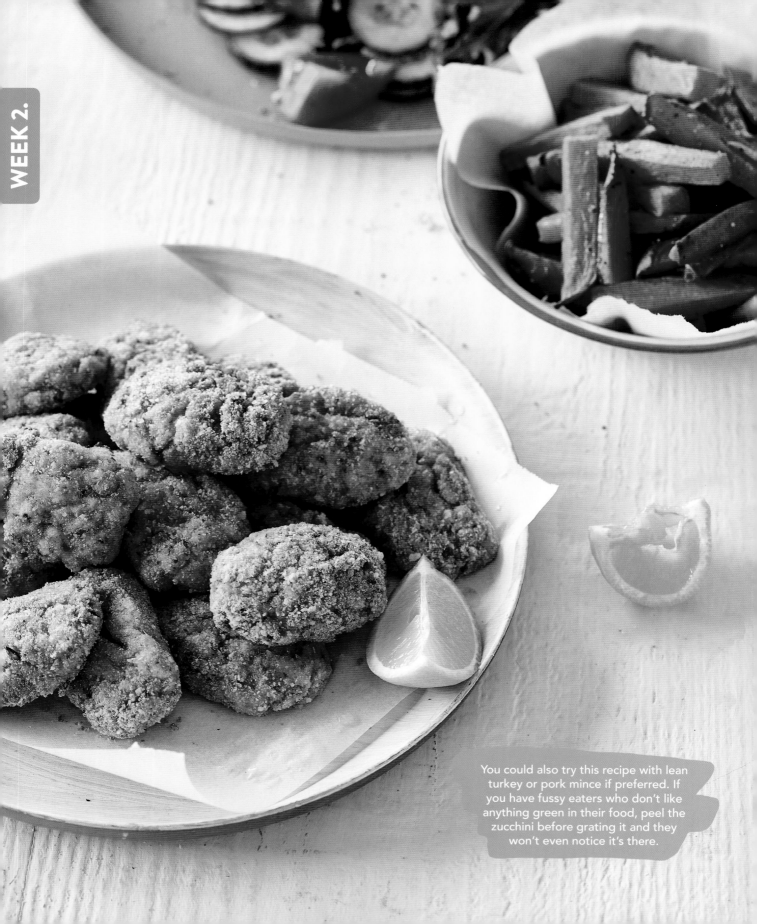

You could also try this recipe with lean turkey or pork mince if preferred. If you have fussy eaters who don't like anything green in their food, peel the zucchini before grating it and they won't even notice it's there.

HIDDEN VEGGIE CHICKEN NUGGETS AND CHIPS

SERVES: 4   **PREPARATION TIME:** 15 MINUTES   **COOKING TIME:** 20 MINUTES

400 g lean chicken mince

1 small zucchini, grated

2 free-range eggs, lightly beaten

salt and freshly ground black pepper

1 cup dried wholemeal breadcrumbs

cooking oil spray

2 small sweet potatoes, cut into chips

120 g mixed lettuce leaves

2 tomatoes, chopped

1 Lebanese cucumber, chopped

lemon wedges, to serve

NUTRI DETAILS PER SERVE

269 cals/1127 kjs

Protein: 30 g

Fibre: 4.6 g

Total fat: 4.5 g

Sat fat: 1.2 g

Carbs: 23.8 g

Total sugar: 7.8 g

Free sugar: 0.0 g

Preheat the oven to 200°C and line a baking tray with baking paper.

Combine the chicken mince, zucchini and egg in a bowl and season well with salt and pepper. Using your hands, press the mixture into bite-sized 'nuggets' and toss to coat in the breadcrumbs. Arrange the nuggets on the prepared tray and spray with cooking oil spray.

Lightly spray a second baking tray with cooking oil spray. Add the sweet potato chips and arrange them in a single layer.

Place the trays in the oven and bake the nuggets for 15–20 minutes or until cooked, and the sweet potato chips for 20 minutes or until tender and golden, turning them both halfway through the cooking time and spraying them lightly with oil again.

Arrange the lettuce, tomato and cucumber on four plates. Add the chicken nuggets and sweet potato chips and serve with lemon wedges.

BEEF RISSOLES WITH VEGGIES

SERVES: 4   **PREPARATION TIME:** 15 MINUTES   **COOKING TIME:** 35 MINUTES

2 small zucchini

2 medium carrots

320 g lean beef mince

⅓ cup rolled oats

2 garlic cloves, crushed

2 free-range eggs, lightly beaten

salt and freshly ground black pepper

2 small sweet potatoes, peeled and diced

⅓ cup reduced-fat milk of choice

200 g cauliflower, cut into florets

2 cups corn kernels (fresh or tinned)

240 g green beans, trimmed

Preheat the oven to 160°C and line a baking tray with baking paper.

Grate the zucchini and carrots into a bowl, then squeeze and drain off any excess liquid. Add the beef mince, oats, garlic and egg and mix well, then season with salt and pepper. Using your hands, shape the mixture into rissoles, making sure you have an equal number for each serve.

Arrange the rissoles on the prepared tray and bake for 35 minutes or until nicely browned and cooked through.

Meanwhile, steam the sweet potato until tender. Remove the pan from the heat, add the milk, season with salt and pepper, and mash until smooth.

Steam the cauliflower, corn and beans until crisp–tender.

Divide the rissoles evenly among four plates and serve with the sweet potato mash and steamed vegetables on the side.

NUTRI DETAILS PER SERVE

400 cals/1674 kjs
Protein: 33 g
Fibre: 9.8 g
Total fat: 11.3 g
Sat fat: 4 g
Carbs: 36.3 g
Total sugar: 12.6 g
Free sugar: 0.0 g

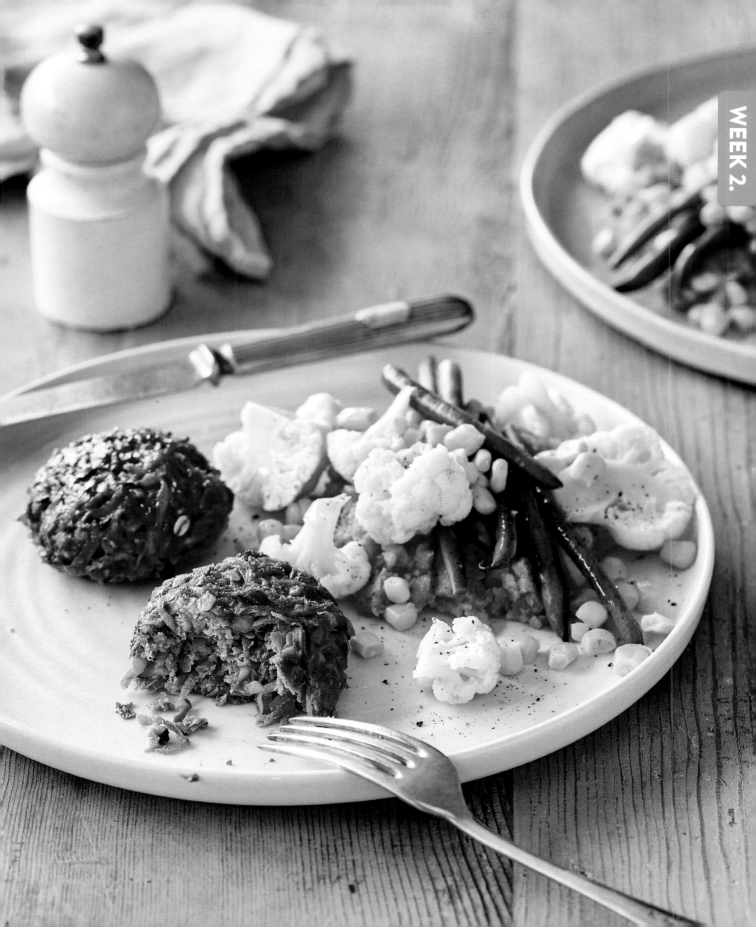

ONE-POT SPAGHETTI BOLOGNESE

SERVES: 6   PREPARATION TIME: 15 MINUTES   COOKING TIME: 30 MINUTES

1 tablespoon extra virgin olive oil

1 red onion, finely diced

2 medium carrots, grated

2 celery stalks, finely chopped

2 garlic cloves, minced

½ bird's eye chilli, finely chopped (optional)

75 g mushrooms, sliced

1 small zucchini, grated

500 g lean beef mince

1 tablespoon worcestershire sauce

3 tablespoons tomato passata

2 × 400 g tins tomatoes

1 cup red wine

2 cups salt-reduced chicken stock

salt and freshly ground black pepper

250 g wholemeal spaghetti

2 tablespoons basil leaves

½ cup shaved parmesan

Heat the olive oil in a large saucepan (it needs to be big enough to hold both the bolognese and the spaghetti) over medium–high heat. Add the onion, carrot, celery and garlic and cook for 3 minutes. Stir in the chilli (if using), then add the mushroom and zucchini and cook for another 2 minutes.

Add the mince to the pan and cook, stirring, for 5 minutes or until the meat is nicely browned, breaking up any lumps with the back of a wooden spoon. Pour in the worcestershire sauce, passata, tomato, wine and stock, season with salt and pepper and stir to combine. Cover with a lid and bring to the boil.

Reduce the heat to medium and remove the lid. Add the spaghetti (you may need to break it in half if your pan isn't big enough) and simmer, stirring regularly, for 15 minutes or until the pasta is al dente.

Divide the spaghetti bolognese among six bowls and sprinkle with the basil and shaved parmesan to serve. Leftovers will keep in an airtight container in the fridge for 3–4 days or in the freezer for up to a month.

NUTRI DETAILS PER SERVE

415 cals/1741 kjs
Protein: 29 g
Fibre: 8 g
Total fat: 13 g
Sat fat: 5 g
Carbs: 34.5 g
Total sugar: 8 g
Free sugar: 0.0 g

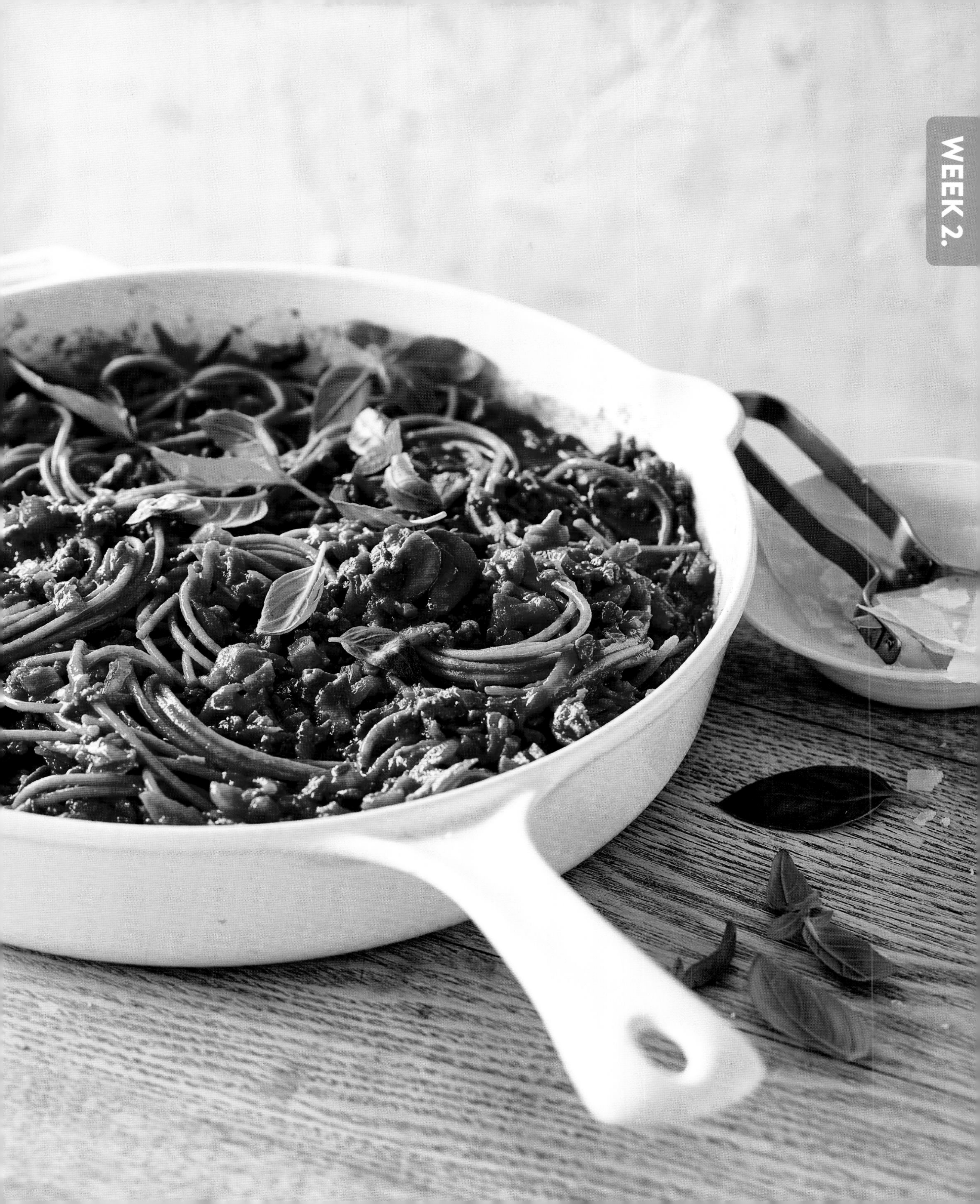

SLOW-COOKED TOFU SAN CHOY BOW

SERVES: 6   **PREPARATION TIME:** 10 MINUTES   **COOKING TIME:** 1 HOUR 35 MINUTES

1 tablespoon sesame oil

2 garlic cloves, minced

2 tablespoons grated ginger

1 brown onion, diced

400 g firm tofu, cut into 2 cm cubes

1 × 400 g tin brown lentils, undrained

2 tablespoons salt-reduced soy sauce

100 g wide rice noodles

12 iceberg lettuce leaves

2 medium carrots, julienned

1 Lebanese cucumber, julienned

⅓ cup unsalted cashews, chopped

NUTRI DETAILS PER SERVE

331 cals/1392 kjs
Protein: 18.7 g
Fibre: 5.3 g
Total fat: 12 g
Sat fat: 1.7 g
Carbs: 32 g
Total sugar: 10.1 g
Free sugar: 0.0 g

Heat the sesame oil in a large heavy-based saucepan or flameproof casserole dish over medium–high heat, add the garlic, ginger and onion and cook for 2–3 minutes or until the onion is translucent.

Add the tofu, lentils (including the liquid from the tin) and soy sauce and stir well. Add 1 cup hot water, then reduce the heat to low and cook, covered, for 1 hour. Remove the lid if the liquid needs to be reduced and cook for another 30 minutes or until the lentils are tender and the mixture has thickened.

Shortly before the lentils are ready, add the rice noodles to a saucepan of boiling water. Reduce the heat and simmer, stirring, for 2–3 minutes or until tender. Drain.

Spoon the noodles into the lettuce leaves and top with the tofu and lentils, carrot and cucumber. Sprinkle with cashews and serve two lettuce cups per person.

Any leftover tofu and lentil mixture can be stored in an airtight container in the fridge for 2–3 days or in the freezer for up to a month.

VARIATION, USING A SLOW-COOKER: Heat the sesame oil in a frying pan over medium–high heat, add the garlic, ginger and onion and cook for 2–3 minutes or until the onion is translucent. Transfer the mixture to a slow cooker. Add the tofu, lentils (including the liquid from the tin) and soy sauce and stir well. Add 1 cup hot water and cook on low for about 4 hours. Remove the lid if the liquid needs to be reduced and cook for another 30 minutes or until the lentils are tender and the mixture has thickened. Prepare the noodles, as above. Spoon the tofu and lentil mixture into the lettuce leaves and top with the noodles, carrot and cucumber. Sprinkle with cashews and serve two lettuce cups per person.

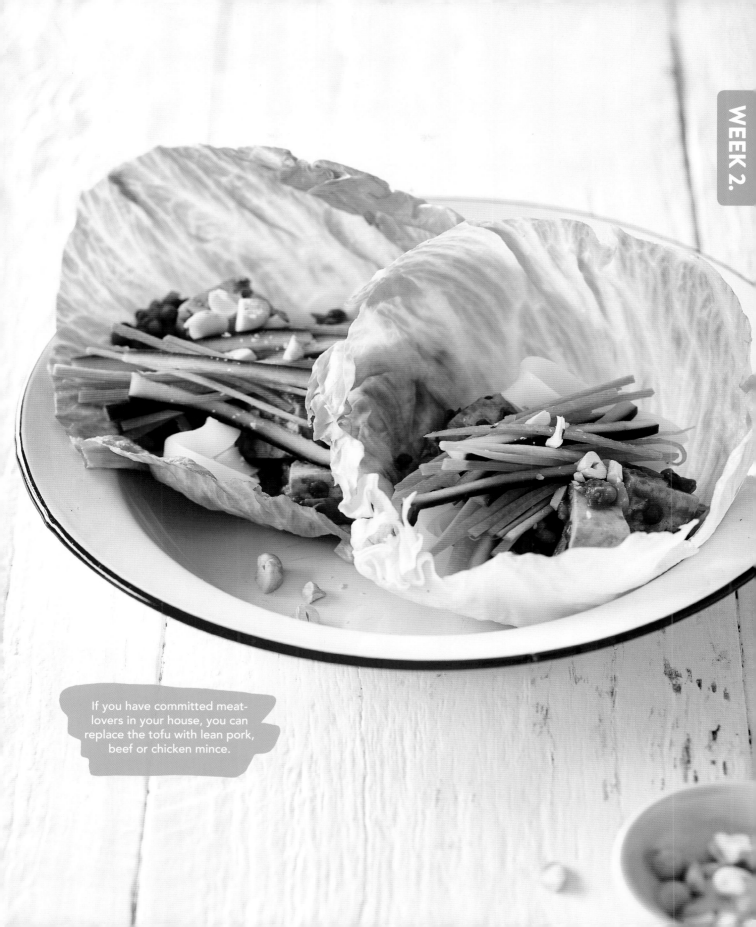

If you have committed meat-lovers in your house, you can replace the tofu with lean pork, beef or chicken mince.

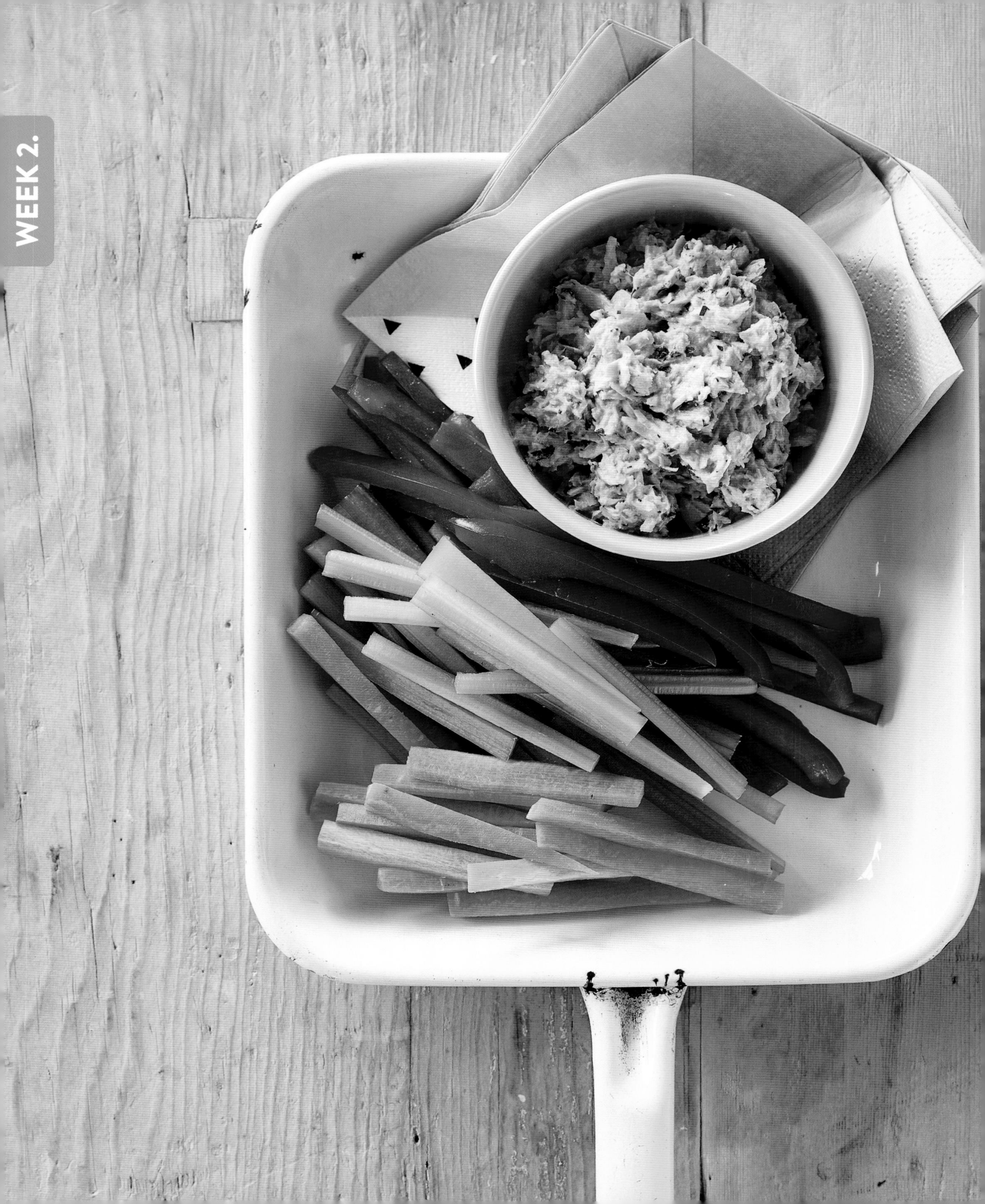

CHILLI TUNA DIP

SERVES: 3   PREPARATION TIME: 10 MINUTES

270 g tinned tuna in spring water, drained

3 tablespoons reduced-fat Greek-style yoghurt

3 teaspoons sweet chilli sauce

3 teaspoons chopped coriander leaves

1 ½ medium carrots, cut into batons

¾ red capsicum, seeds removed, cut into batons

3 celery stalks, cut into batons

Place the tuna, yoghurt, chilli sauce and coriander in a bowl and mix until well combined.

Divide the dip and vegetable dippers into three portions and serve. Any leftover dip and veggie sticks will keep in an airtight container in the fridge for 2–3 days.

NUTRI DETAILS PER SERVE

160 cals/671 kjs
Protein: 23.4 g
Fibre: 2.2 g
Total fat: 2.8 g
Sat fat: 1 g
Carbs: 7.7 g
Total sugar: 7.3 g
Free sugar: 3 g

SWEET POTATO AND CHAMOMILE CRACKERS

SERVES: 3 **PREPARATION TIME:** 15 MINUTES **COOKING TIME:** 50 MINUTES

¾ cup rolled oats

1 ½ small sweet potatoes, peeled and cut into chunks

1 chamomile teabag

1 ½ tablespoons coconut oil, melted

1 ½ tablespoons reduced-fat Greek-style yoghurt

NUTRI DETAILS PER SERVE

178 cals/748 kjs
Protein: 6.6 g
Fibre: 4.5 g
Total fat: 10.5 g
Sat fat: 7.1 g
Carbs: 12.3 g
Total sugar: 5.5 g
Free sugar: 0.0 g

Preheat the oven to 180°C and line a baking tray with baking paper.

Place the oats in a food processor and blitz to form a fine flour (you could also use pre-made oat flour if you prefer).

Place the sweet potato in a saucepan, cover with water and bring to the boil. Add the teabag and boil for 10–12 minutes or until the sweet potato is tender. Remove the teabag and drain, reserving 1–2 teaspoons of the cooking liquid.

Place the sweet potato and reserved cooking liquid in a food processor and process on high until smooth. Transfer to a bowl, add the oat flour and coconut oil and mix well to combine.

Transfer the dough to the prepared tray and roll out to approximately 5 mm thick. Score the dough into 12 crackers and bake for 15–20 minutes.

Remove from the oven and carefully slide the baking paper off the tray. Reline the tray with a fresh piece of baking paper. Flip the crackers over onto the new sheet of paper, then peel off the original paper and return the crackers to the oven for another 10–15 minutes or until golden and crisp.

Break into individual crackers and serve four crackers per person with yoghurt for dipping.

Leftover crackers will keep in an airtight container in the pantry for 3–4 days.

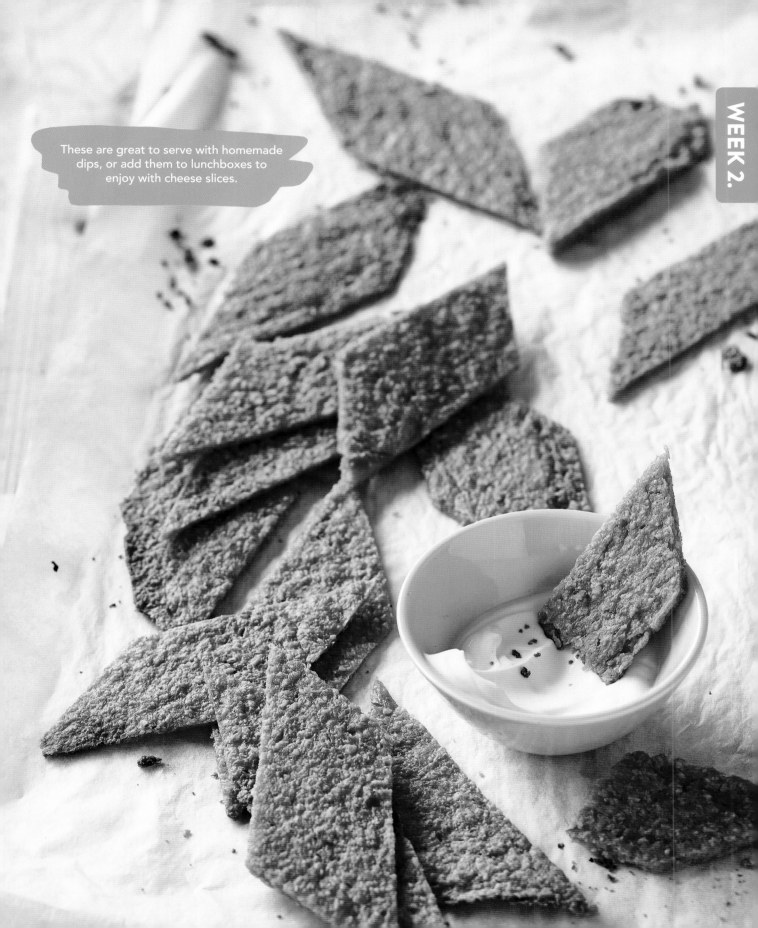

These are great to serve with homemade dips, or add them to lunchboxes to enjoy with cheese slices.

CHOCOLATE MUESLI BARS

SERVES: 8   PREPARATION TIME: 5 MINUTES, PLUS CHILLING TIME   COOKING TIME: 5 MINUTES

½ cup coconut oil
3 tablespoons pure maple syrup
½ cup cacao/cocoa powder
1 cup untoasted muesli

NUTRI DETAILS PER SERVE

197 cals/829 kjs
Protein: 2.3 g
Fibre: 1.9 g
Total fat: 14.3 g
Sat fat: 12.7 g
Carbs: 14.8 g
Total sugar: 8.5 g
Free sugar: 6 g

Line a 20 cm square cake tin or container with baking paper and set aside.

Place the coconut oil and maple syrup in a saucepan and heat until warm and melted. Remove from the heat and add the cacao/cocoa powder, stirring quickly to combine and smooth out any lumps. Mix in the muesli, making sure it is evenly coated in the chocolate mixture.

Pour the muesli mixture into the prepared tin and chill in the fridge for 1 hour or until firm.

Cut into eight bars. Leftovers will keep in an airtight container in the fridge for up to 2 weeks or in the freezer for a month.

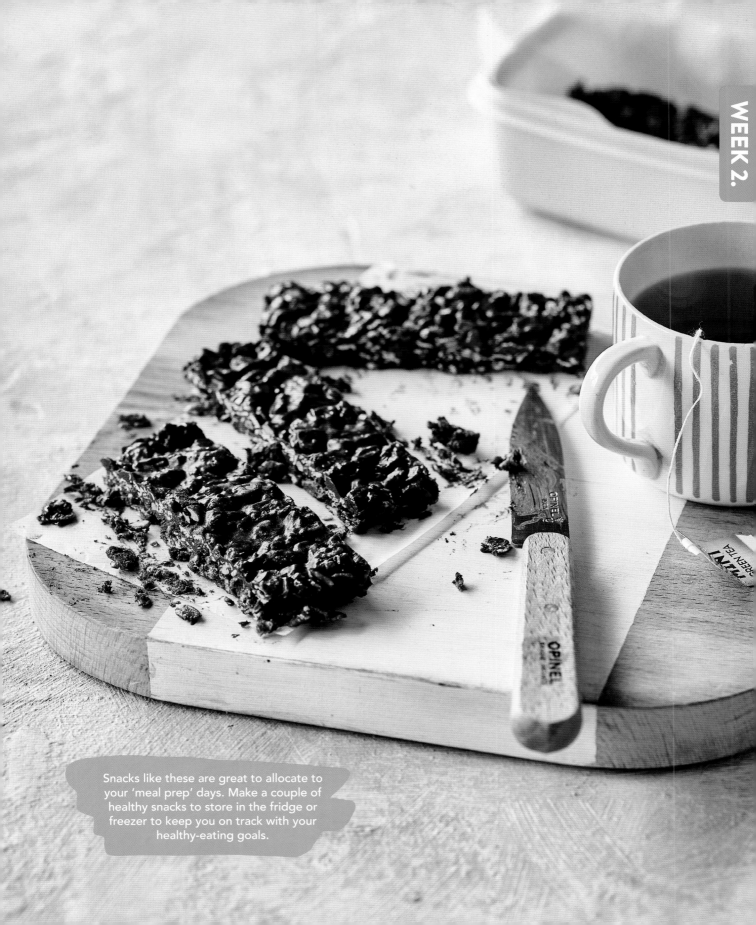

Snacks like these are great to allocate to your 'meal prep' days. Make a couple of healthy snacks to store in the fridge or freezer to keep you on track with your healthy-eating goals.

Place the coconut cream in the fridge overnight and use the thick, extra creamy part that settles on the top for this recipe. The coconut water that separates from the cream is great in a smoothie or may be frozen to use another time. You can also freeze any leftover thick coconut cream in ice-cube trays to use in other recipes.

CHOC-MINT CREAMS

SERVES: 4 PREPARATION TIME: 10 MINUTES, PLUS CHILLING TIME COOKING TIME: 5 MINUTES

⅓ cup coconut cream, chilled
1 teaspoon peppermint extract
1 teaspoon pure maple syrup
½ teaspoon vanilla extract
20 squares (about 100 g) dark
    chocolate (70% cocoa solids)

NUTRI DETAILS PER SERVE

171 cals/717 kjs
Protein: 1.4 g
Fibre: 1.5 g
Total fat: 11.5 g
Sat fat: 10.3 g
Carbs: 16 g
Total sugar: 15.5 g
Free sugar: 14.8 g

Place the coconut cream, peppermint extract, maple syrup and vanilla in a bowl and mix to combine. Pour into eight silicone mini muffin moulds. (Silicone works best but you could also line a regular mini muffin tin with paper cases or baking paper for easy removal.)

Place the moulds in the freezer for 1½ hours or until the mint cream has set.

Break the chocolate into squares and melt in a small heatproof bowl set over a saucepan of simmering water, stirring occasionally. Set aside to cool slightly.

Gently remove the frozen mint creams from the moulds and, using a toothpick, quickly dip them in the chocolate, coating the bottom. Place on a tray or plate lined with baking paper, with the chocolate side facing down. Spoon the remaining melted chocolate over the mint creams to cover the top and sides. Refrigerate for 30 minutes or until the chocolate is set.

One serve is two choc-mint creams. You can make a larger batch of these if you like and store them in the freezer or in an airtight container in the fridge for 4–5 days. Eat them straight from the freezer or let them thaw and soften for 10 minutes first.

CHEESY BROCCOLI BITES

SERVES: 4   PREPARATION TIME: 10 MINUTES   COOKING TIME: 15 MINUTES

200 g broccoli, cut into florets
2 free-range eggs
½ cup dried wholemeal
  breadcrumbs
½ cup grated parmesan
2 tablespoons coconut oil

NUTRI DETAILS PER SERVE

154 cals/646 kjs
Protein: 7.4 g
Fibre: 1.4 g
Total fat: 10.5 g
Sat fat: 2.9 g
Carbs: 7 g
Total sugar: 0.6 g
Free sugar: 0.0 g

Steam the broccoli or cook in the microwave for about 3 minutes until bright green and just tender. Cool slightly, then blitz in a food processor to form fine crumbs.

Tip the broccoli crumbs into a medium bowl, add the egg, breadcrumbs and parmesan and stir well. Use your hands to form the mixture into 16 balls.

Melt half the coconut oil in a frying pan over medium heat. Add half the balls and gently press the tops to flatten a little. Cook for 2–3 minutes on each side until golden. Remove and drain on paper towel, then repeat with the remaining coconut oil and balls.

Serve four broccoli bites per person. Any leftovers will keep in an airtight container in the fridge for 3–4 days. They can be served hot or cold.

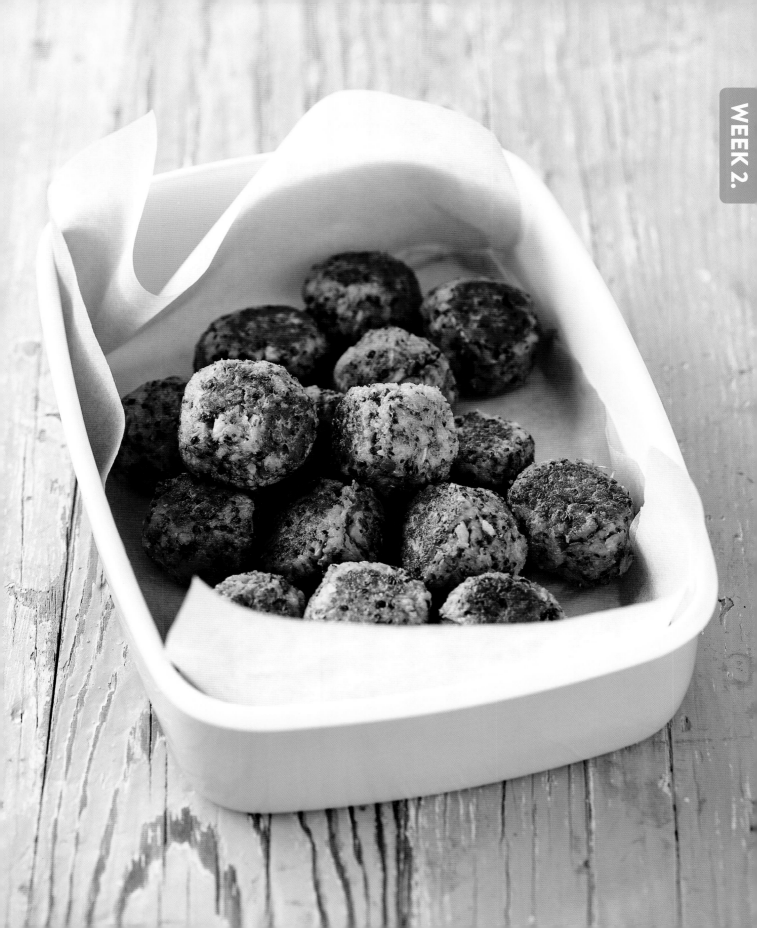

WEEK 3.

MEAL & EXERCISE PLAN

	MONDAY	TUESDAY	WEDNESDAY
BREAKFAST	Banoffee Breakfast Bowl **p.146** 398 cals	Chocolate Chia Breakfast Muffins **p.148** 213 cals	Feta, Tomato and Spinach Toastie **p.151** 297 cals
MORNING SNACK	Sesame and Sweet Potato Dip **p.188** 148 cals	Spinach Balls **p.190** 267 cals	½ cup Greek-style yoghurt with ½ cup mixed berries 147 cals
LUNCH	Caramelised Pear with Turkey and Rocket Salad **p.161** 308 cals	Barbecue Beef Wrap **p.162** 241 cals	Creamy Chicken and Corn Soup **p.164** 253 cals
EXERCISE	20 Minute Metabolic Booster**, Workout 1 (see page 284)	20 minute Body Strong Pilates, Workout 1 (see page 286)	20 minute Deep Core Conditioning*, Workout 1 (see page 290)
AFTERNOON SNACK	1 orange served with 1 cup herbal tea 54 cals	Cherry-Choc Slice **p.193** 253 cals	Paprika Parmesan Chips **p.194** 115 cals
DINNER	Marinated Salmon with Quinoa and Roast Vegetable Salad **p.174** 416 cals	Bacon, Spinach and Tomato Risotto **p.177** 338 cals	Tandoori Lamb with Couscous Salad **p.178** 449 cals
EVENING SNACK	½ cup Greek-style yoghurt with ½ cup mixed berries 147 cals	Blueberry Mousse with Pistachios **p.196** 187 cals	Blueberry Mousse with Pistachios **p.196** 187 cals
TOTAL CALORIES	**1471 cals**	**1499 cals**	**1448 cals**

** Choose the low-impact 20 Minute Tummy Tamer workout to complete today if you are still recovering from a C-section, abdominal separation, prolapse, or if you have a weak pelvic floor.

THURSDAY	FRIDAY	SATURDAY	SUNDAY
Onion and Cheese Omelette p.152 269 cals	Sweet Potato Toast with Scrambled Egg and Tomato p.154 288 cals	White Bean Pancakes with Strawberries and Passionfruit p.156 414 cals	Corn Fritters with Avocado Salsa p.158 386 cals
Spinach Balls p.190 267 cals	Sesame and Sweet Potato Dip p.188 148 cals	Paprika Parmesan Chips p.194 115 cals	1 orange served with 1 cup herbal tea 54 cals
Tuna and Citrus Salad p.166 289 cals	Chicken Pasta Caesar Salad p.169 368 cals	Crustless Quiches p.170 277 cals	Green Mac and Cheese p.172 318 cals
14 minute Total Body Tabata Workout (see page 296)	**20 minute Butt and Thigh*, Workout 1 (see page 298)**	**20 minute Fat Blaster, Workout 1 (see page 302)**	**Active Recovery Day 1 (see page 304)**
Paprika Parmesan Chips p.194 115 cals	1 orange served with 1 cup of herbal tea 54 cals	Sesame and Sweet Potato Dip p.188 148 cals	Sesame and Sweet Potato Dip p.188 148 cals
Quick Chicken Laksa p.180 390 cals	Greek Beef Burgers p.182 405 cals	Naked Chicken Parma with Popcorn Cauliflower p.185 396 cals	Lentil and Quinoa Salad with Eggs and Pesto p.186 407 cals
½ cup Greek-style yoghurt with ½ cup mixed berries 147 cals	Blueberry Mousse with Pistachios p.196 187 cals	1 orange served with 1 cup herbal tea 54 cals	½ cup Greek-style yoghurt with ½ cup mixed berries 147 cals
1477 cals	**1450 cals**	**1404 cals**	**1460 cals**

*Choose the low-impact variation of this workout if you are still recovering from a C-section, abdominal separation, prolapse, or if you have a weak pelvic floor.

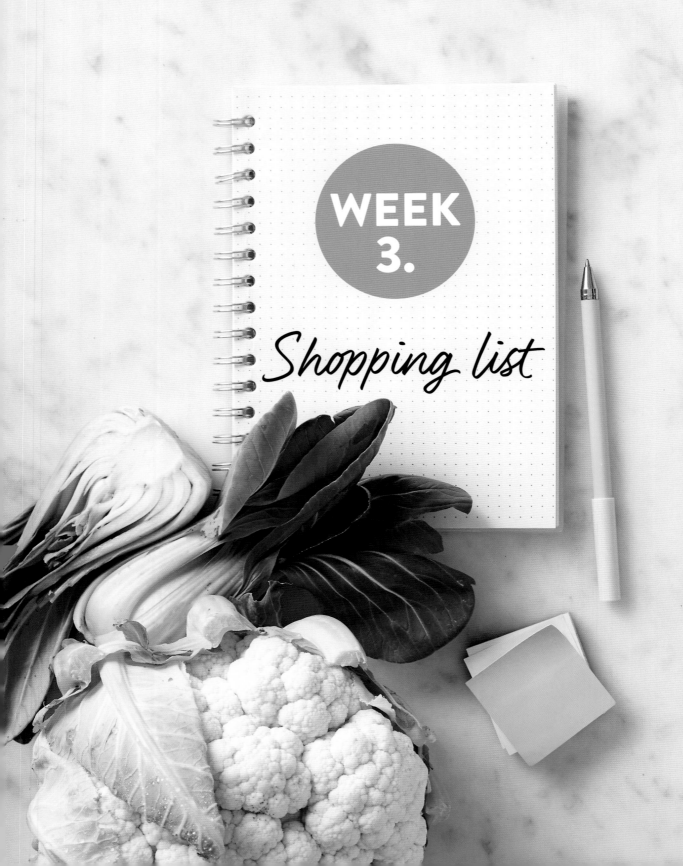

WEEK
3.

Shopping list

Vegetables

Baby spinach leaves 210 g
Bok choy (4) 600 g
Capsicum, red 1
Carrots 2
Cauliflower 400 g
Celery 1 stalk
Corn kernels 800 g (or used tinned)
Cucumber, Lebanese 2
Garlic 3 cloves
Ginger 1 small knob
Kale 60 g
Lettuce, cos 60 g
Lettuce, mixed leaves 210 g
Onions, brown 2
Onions, red 2
Radishes 2
Rocket leaves 180 g
Spring onions 7
Sweet potatoes, small 3
Tomatoes 10
Zucchini 3

Fruit

Avocado 1
Banana 1
Blueberries 200 g (or use frozen)
Cherries 150 g (or use frozen)
Grapefruit 1
Lemons 5
Lime 1
Oranges 5
Passionfruit 1
Pears 2
Strawberries 65 g

Fresh herbs

Basil 1 bunch
Chives 1 bunch
Coriander 1 bunch
Flat-leaf parsley 2 bunches
Mint 2 bunches

Meat, fish and poultry

Bacon rashers, lean and trimmed (6) 165 g
Beef mince, lean 320 g
Beef steak, lean 140 g
Chicken breast fillets 1.3 kg
Eggs, free range 20
Ham, smoked, lean 40 g (2 slices)
Lamb cutlets (8) about 480 g
Salmon fillet (or firm fish of choice) 400 g
Turkey, smoked, lean, sliced 120 g

Dairy and soy

Cheddar, reduced-fat grated 235 g
Feta, reduced-fat 160 g
Mozzarella, reduced-fat 50 g
Tofu, silken 100 g
Yoghurt, reduced-fat natural
    Greek-style 365 g

Breads, grains, cereals and nuts

Bread of choice, wholemeal
    or gluten free, 5 slices
Bread rolls, wholegrain 4
Tortillas, wholemeal 6

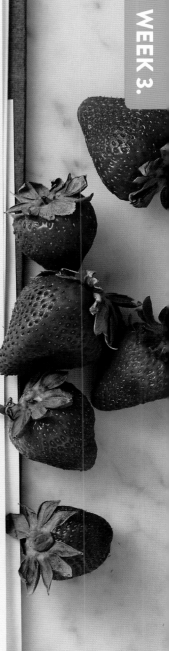

BANOFFEE BREAKFAST BOWL

SERVES: 2   **PREPARATION TIME:** 10 MINUTES   **COOKING TIME:** 5 MINUTES

½ cup pitted dried dates, chopped

1 cup reduced-fat milk of choice

1 cup rolled oats

⅓ cup reduced-fat Greek-style yoghurt

2 teaspoons honey

1 small banana, sliced

1 tablespoon crushed peanuts

Place the dates, milk and ½ cup water in a saucepan over low heat for 5 minutes or until the dates are softened. Allow to cool slightly, then place in a food processor with the oats and process on high to form a smooth puree.

Divide the puree between two bowls. Top with the yoghurt, honey, banana and peanuts, and serve.

NUTRI DETAILS PER SERVE

398 cals/1667 kjs
Protein: 18.5 g
Fibre: 11.4 g
Total fat: 9.8 g
Sat fat: 2.5 g
Carbs: 53 g
Total sugar: 48 g
Free sugar: 8 g

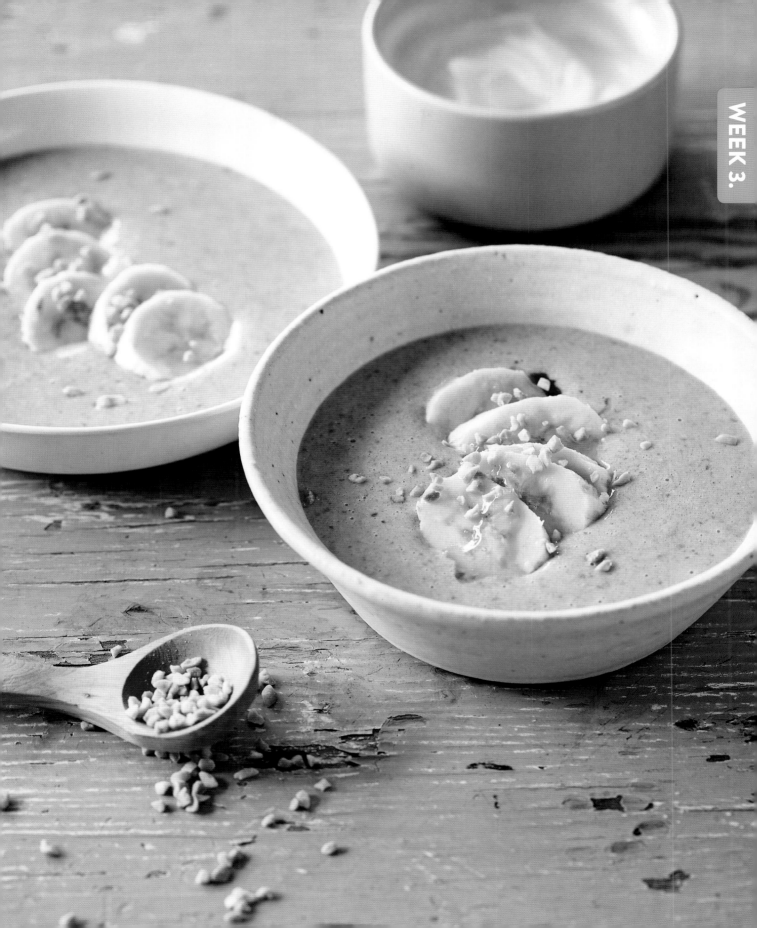

CHOCOLATE CHIA BREAKFAST MUFFINS

SERVES: 12   **PREPARATION TIME:** 10 MINUTES, PLUS STANDING TIME   **COOKING TIME:** 25 MINUTES

1 cup reduced-fat milk of choice
3 tablespoons chia seeds
½ cup honey
125 g butter, softened
1 cup spelt flour
½ cup plain wholemeal flour
2 tablespoons cacao/cocoa powder
2 teaspoons baking powder

NUTRI DETAILS PER SERVE

213 cals/896 kjs
Protein: 4.4 g
Fibre: 3 g
Total fat: 10.6 g
Sat fat: 6.1 g
Carbs: 24.6 g
Total sugar: 13.6 g
Free sugar: 11.3 g

Preheat the oven to 180°C. Line a 12-hole standard muffin tin with baking paper or patty pan cases.

Combine the milk and chia seeds in a bowl, then set aside for about 20 minutes to allow the chia seeds to absorb the milk. Stir regularly to prevent the seeds from sinking to the bottom.

Meanwhile, place the honey and butter in a bowl and mix with a wooden spoon until combined and smooth. Add the milk and chia seed mixture and combine well.

Sift in the spelt and wholemeal flours, cacao/cocoa powder and baking powder and mix just to combine. Don't overmix the batter or the muffins will be tough.

Spoon the batter evenly into the muffin holes and bake for 20–25 minutes or until a skewer inserted in the centre comes out clean. Cool in the tin for 5 minutes then serve warm, or turn them out onto a wire rack to cool completely.

One serve is one muffin. Store leftovers in an airtight container in the fridge for 3–4 days or in the freezer for up to 3 months.

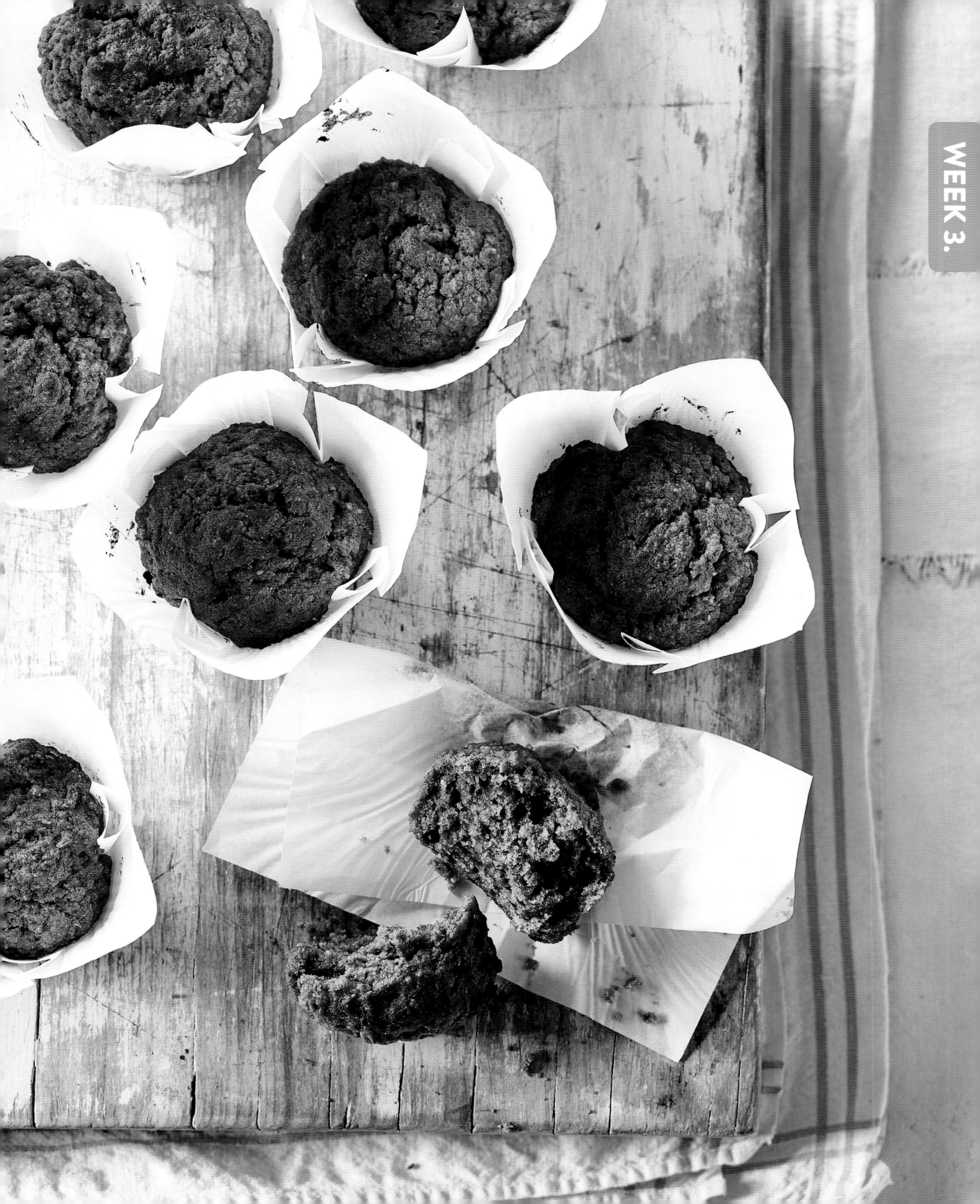

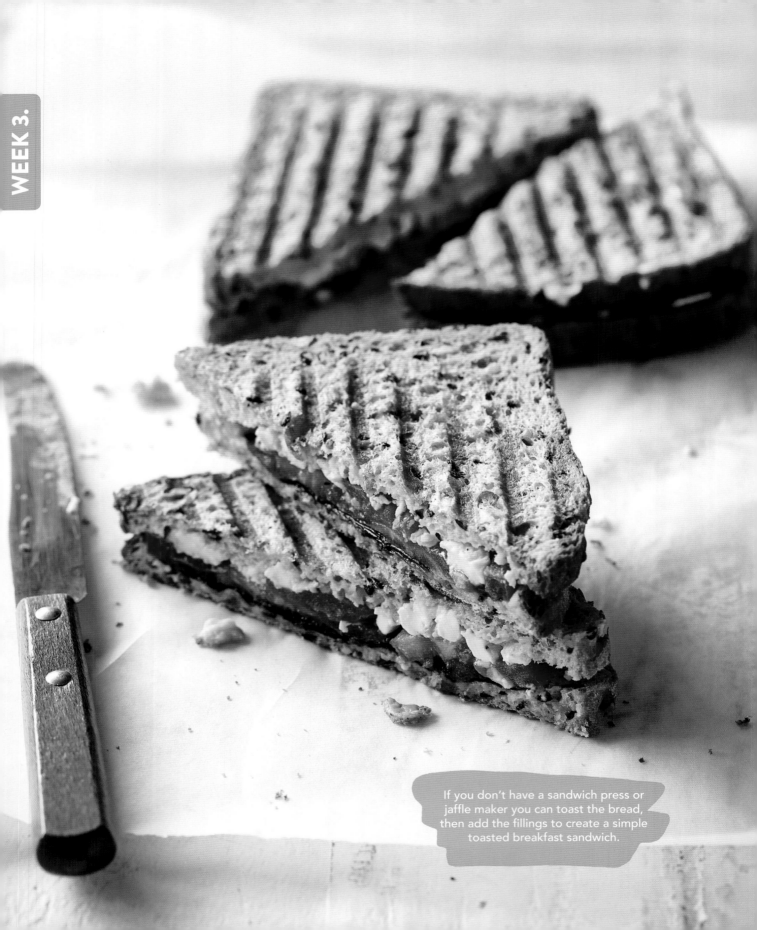

If you don't have a sandwich press or jaffle maker you can toast the bread, then add the fillings to create a simple toasted breakfast sandwich.

FETA, TOMATO AND SPINACH TOASTIE

SERVES: 2   **PREPARATION TIME:** 5 MINUTES   **COOKING TIME:** 5 MINUTES

4 slices wholegrain or gluten-free bread of choice
1 tomato, sliced
freshly ground black pepper
80 g reduced-fat feta, crumbled
30 g baby spinach leaves
½ teaspoon extra virgin olive oil

Preheat a sandwich press or jaffle maker.

Place two slices of bread on a board and top with the tomato, pepper, feta and baby spinach leaves. Drizzle with a little olive oil and sandwich with the remaining slices of bread.

Cook in a sandwich press or jaffle maker until the bread is golden and the cheese has melted.

NUTRI DETAILS PER SERVE

297 cals/1248 kjs
Protein: 18.8 g
Fibre: 6 g
Total fat: 9.3 g
Sat fat: 4.2 g
Carbs: 31.4 g
Total sugar: 2.9 g
Free sugar: 0.0 g

ONION AND CHEESE OMELETTE

SERVES: 2   **PREPARATION TIME:** 5 MINUTES   **COOKING TIME:** 15 MINUTES

2 teaspoons extra virgin olive oil

½ red onion, sliced

10 g butter

4 free-range eggs

½ cup grated reduced-fat cheddar

2 tablespoons chopped chives

NUTRI DETAILS PER SERVE

269 cals/1129 kjs
Protein: 20.8 g
Fibre: 0.2 g
Total fat: 19 g
Sat fat: 7 g
Carbs: 0.8 g
Total sugar: 0.7 g
Free sugar: 0.0 g

Heat the olive oil in a frying pan over medium–high heat. Reduce the heat to medium, add the onion and cook for 2–3 minutes or until soft and golden. Remove the onion to a plate.

Melt half the butter in the pan. Lightly beat two of the eggs, add to the pan and swirl to cover the base. Sprinkle half the onion, cheese and chives over the egg, then cover the pan with a lid and cook for 5–7 minutes or until the egg is just cooked through and the cheese has melted. Fold the omelette in half and keep warm while you repeat with the remaining ingredients to make a second omelette. Serve immediately.

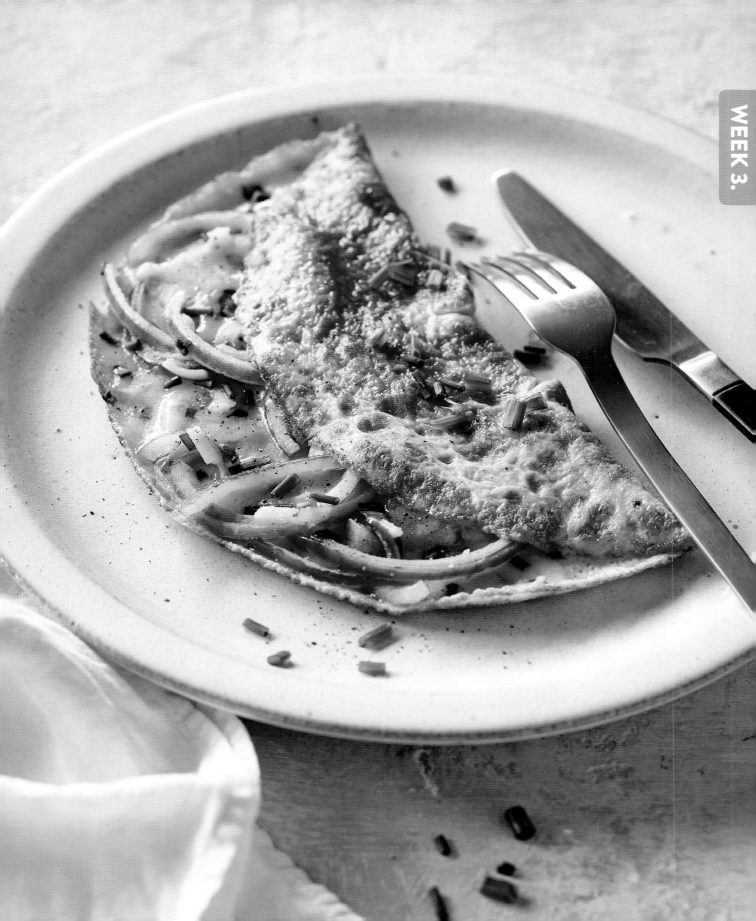

SWEET POTATO TOAST WITH SCRAMBLED EGG AND TOMATO

SERVES: 2   **PREPARATION TIME:** 10 MINUTES   **COOKING TIME:** 10 MINUTES

4 free-range eggs

2 tablespoons reduced-fat milk of choice

cooking oil spray

2 small sweet potatoes, each cut lengthways into 4 slices

60 g rocket leaves

1 tomato, chopped

freshly ground black pepper

NUTRI DETAILS PER SERVE

288 cals/1203 kjs
Protein: 19 g
Fibre: 6.1 g
Total fat: 9.6 g
Sat fat: 2.8 g
Carbs: 28.2 g
Total sugar: 14.5 g
Free sugar: 0.0 g

Beat together the eggs and milk in a bowl.

Spray a medium frying pan with cooking oil spray and place over medium heat. Add the egg mixture and gently scrape across the pan with a flat spatula until the egg is cooked and scrambled.

Meanwhile, place the sweet potato slices in a toaster or place them under a preheated overhead grill and toast until golden and tender.

Divide the sweet potato toast between two plates and top with the rocket, scrambled egg and tomato. Season with pepper and serve.

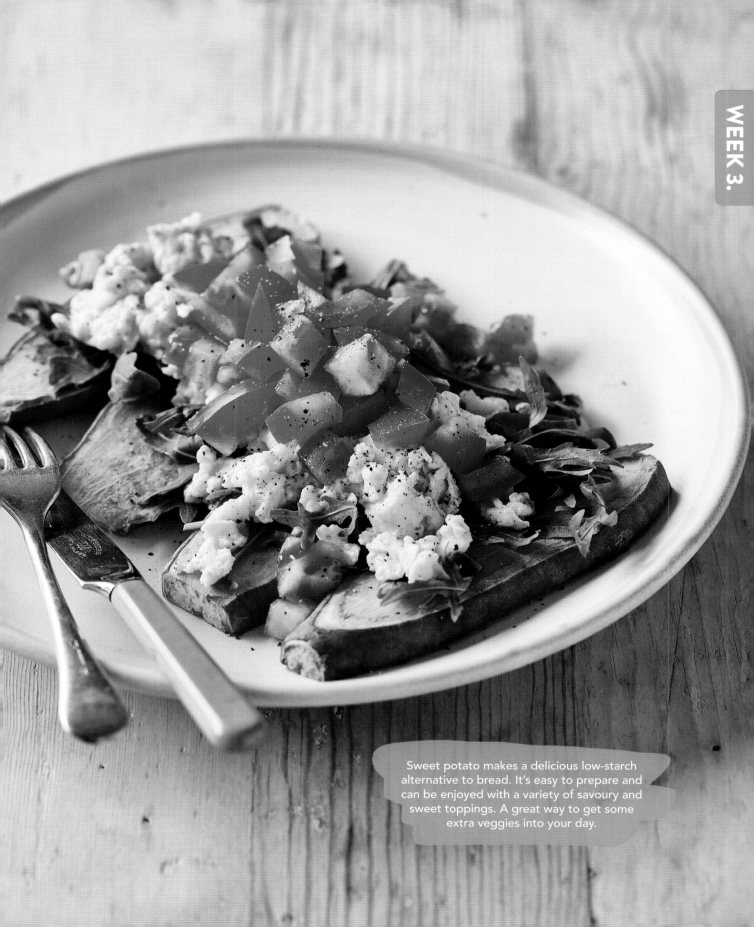

Sweet potato makes a delicious low-starch alternative to bread. It's easy to prepare and can be enjoyed with a variety of savoury and sweet toppings. A great way to get some extra veggies into your day.

WHITE BEAN PANCAKES WITH STRAWBERRIES AND PASSIONFRUIT

SERVES: 2   **PREPARATION TIME:** 10 MINUTES, PLUS STANDING TIME   **COOKING TIME:** 12 MINUTES

- 100 g tinned cannellini beans, drained and rinsed
- 1 free-range egg
- ½ teaspoon vanilla extract
- 1 cup wholemeal self-raising flour
- ¾ cup reduced-fat milk of choice
- 65 g strawberries, sliced
- 1 tablespoon passionfruit pulp
- 1 tablespoon pure maple syrup

Place the cannellini beans in a food processor and process on high until smooth. Add the egg and vanilla and process until well combined. Transfer to a bowl and add the flour, then whisk in the milk to form a smooth batter. Set aside for 10 minutes.

Heat a large non-stick frying pan over medium–high heat, add 3 tablespoons of the batter for each pancake and cook for 3 minutes or until bubbles start to form on the surface. Flip and cook for a further minute or until light golden. Repeat to make four pancakes in total.

Place two pancakes on each plate and top with the sliced strawberries and passionfruit pulp. Finish with a drizzle of maple syrup and serve.

NUTRI DETAILS PER SERVE

414 cals/1733 kjs
Protein: 16.7 g
Fibre: 12.1 g
Total fat: 5.1 g
Sat fat: 1.7 g
Carbs: 68.7 g
Total sugar: 25 g
Free sugar: 7.9 g

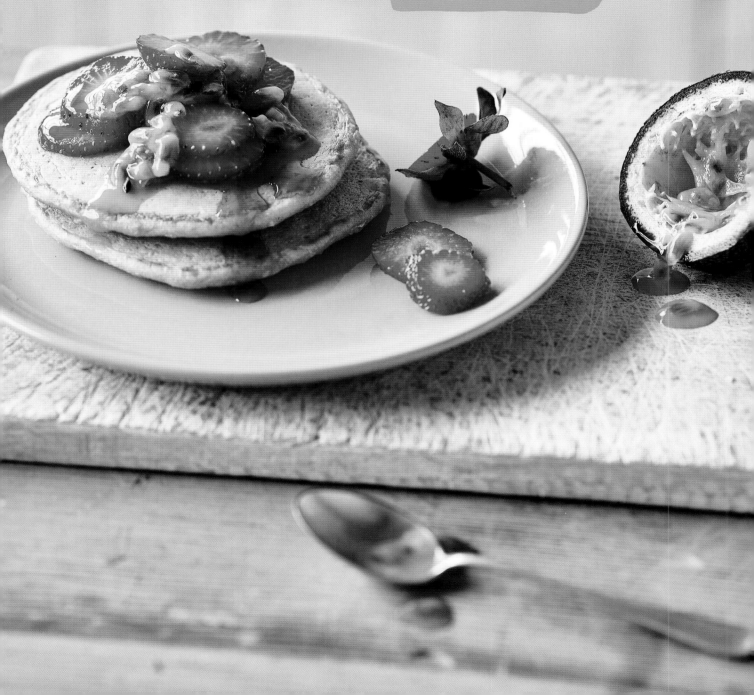

You can make a larger batch of this pancake batter and store it in an airtight container in the fridge for 1–2 days. Repeating meals on consecutive days will save you time and money.

CORN FRITTERS WITH AVOCADO SALSA

SERVES: 2   PREPARATION TIME: 10 MINUTES   COOKING TIME: 15 MINUTES

- 2 cups corn kernels (fresh or tinned)
- 2 free-range eggs, lightly beaten
- 1 tablespoon cornflour
- 1 tablespoon plain wholemeal flour
- 2 spring onions, finely chopped
- ⅓ cup chopped flat-leaf parsley leaves
- salt and freshly ground black pepper
- cooking oil spray
- ½ medium avocado, diced
- 2 teaspoons lime juice, plus extra if needed
- ¼ red onion, finely diced
- ⅓ cup finely chopped coriander leaves
- 2 teaspoons sweet chilli sauce, plus extra if needed

Combine the corn, egg, cornflour, flour, spring onion and parsley in a bowl and season with salt and pepper.

Spray a large frying pan with cooking oil spray and place over medium heat. Add 2 tablespoons of the batter for each fritter and cook for 3–4 minutes each side or until golden and cooked through. Be careful not to heat the pan too much as you want the fritters to cook all the way through without burning on the outside.

Remove the fritters and drain on paper towel, then repeat with the remaining mixture to make 2–3 fritters per serve.

Meanwhile, combine the avocado, lime juice, red onion, coriander and sweet chilli sauce in a bowl. Taste and adjust the lime juice and sweet chilli sauce if required. Season with a little salt.

Divide the fritters evenly between two plates, top with a dollop of avocado salsa and serve.

NUTRI DETAILS PER SERVE

386 cals/1616 kjs
Protein: 13 g
Fibre: 7.2 g
Total fat: 16 g
Sat fat: 4 g
Carbs: 43 g
Total sugar: 8.9 g
Free sugar: 1.5 g

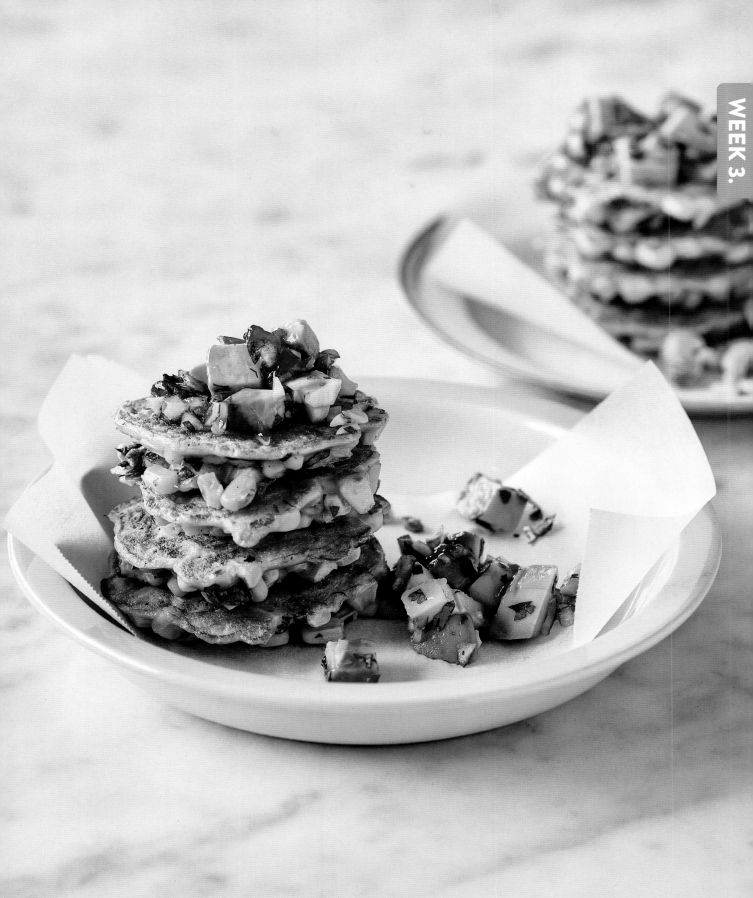

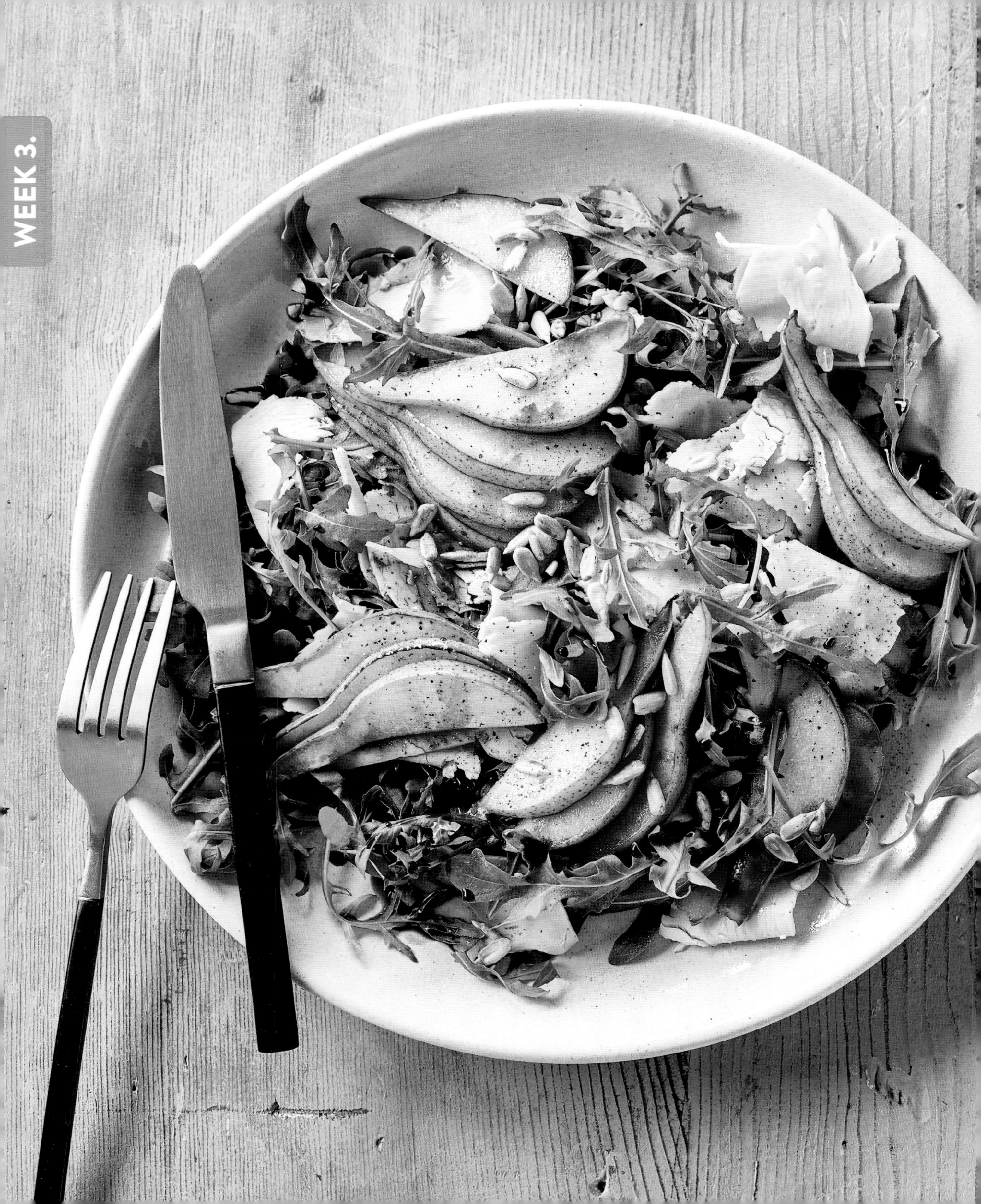

CARAMELISED PEAR WITH TURKEY AND ROCKET SALAD

SERVES: 2   **PREPARATION TIME:** 5 MINUTES   **COOKING TIME:** 5 MINUTES

2 tablespoons sunflower seeds
2 teaspoons extra virgin olive oil
2 pears, cored and sliced
2 teaspoons honey
120 g rocket leaves
120 g lean smoked turkey, torn
2 tablespoons balsamic vinegar

NUTRI DETAILS PER SERVE

308 cals/1294 kjs
Protein: 20 g
Fibre: 6 g
Total fat: 14.2 g
Sat fat: 1.8 g
Carbs: 26.3 g
Total sugar: 18 g
Free sugar: 5.8 g

Roast the sunflower seeds in a dry frying pan over low heat, then set aside.

Heat the olive oil in the same pan over medium heat, add the pear slices and cook for 3 minutes or until the pear is golden brown on both sides. Drizzle the honey over the pear, then remove from the heat and set aside.

Divide the rocket between two plates and top with the caramelised pear, turkey and sunflower seeds. Drizzle with balsamic vinegar and serve.

BARBECUE BEEF WRAP

SERVES: 2   **PREPARATION TIME:** 10 MINUTES   **COOKING TIME:** 5 MINUTES

140 g lean beef steak
cooking oil spray
2 wholemeal tortillas
30 g mixed lettuce leaves
½ tomato, sliced
1 medium carrot, grated
2 teaspoons barbecue sauce
(with no added sugar)

Cut the beef into thin strips and tenderise using a meat mallet or the base of a heavy saucepan.

Lightly spray a frying pan with cooking oil spray and place over high heat. Add the beef and cook, stirring, for 2 minutes or until browned and cooked through. Remove from the heat and set aside.

Top the tortillas with the lettuce, tomato, carrot and beef, and finish with a drizzle of barbecue sauce. Roll up to enclose the filling and serve.

NUTRI DETAILS PER SERVE

241 cals/1009 kjs
Protein: 20.2 g
Fibre: 4.8 g
Total fat: 5.1 g
Sat fat: 1.6 g
Carbs: 25.8 g
Total sugar: 5.7 g
Free sugar: 0.0 g

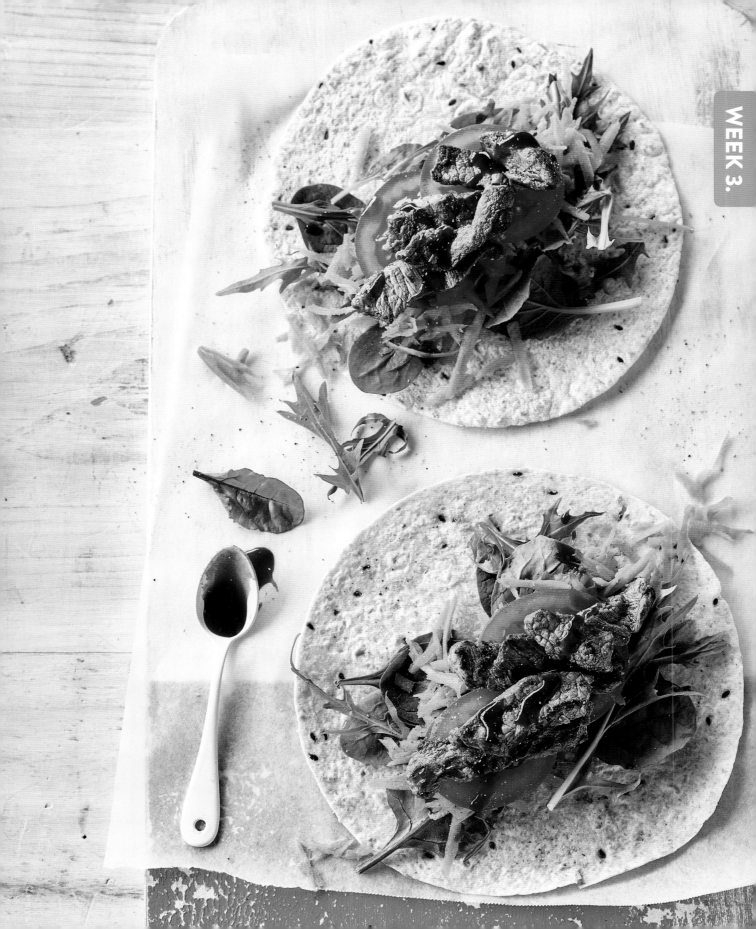

CREAMY CHICKEN AND CORN SOUP

SERVES: 2   PREPARATION TIME: 10 MINUTES   COOKING TIME: 10 MINUTES

---

2 cups corn kernels (fresh or tinned)

1 cup salt-reduced chicken stock

1 cup reduced-fat milk of choice

200 g chicken breast fillets, cut into thin strips

1 teaspoon salt-reduced soy sauce

1 spring onion, shredded

Place the corn in a food processor and pulse until roughly chopped. Transfer the corn to a medium saucepan, add the stock and milk and bring to the boil over medium–high heat.

Add the chicken strips to the hot soup. Reduce the heat to medium and simmer for 3–4 minutes or until the chicken is cooked through.

Ladle the soup into two bowls and drizzle over the soy sauce. Garnish with spring onion and serve.

NUTRI DETAILS PER SERVE

253 cals/1060 kjs
Protein: 31.3 g
Fibre: 2.3 g
Total fat: 3.6 g
Sat fat: 0.9 g
Carbs: 23.1 g
Total sugar: 10.9 g
Free sugar: 0.0 g

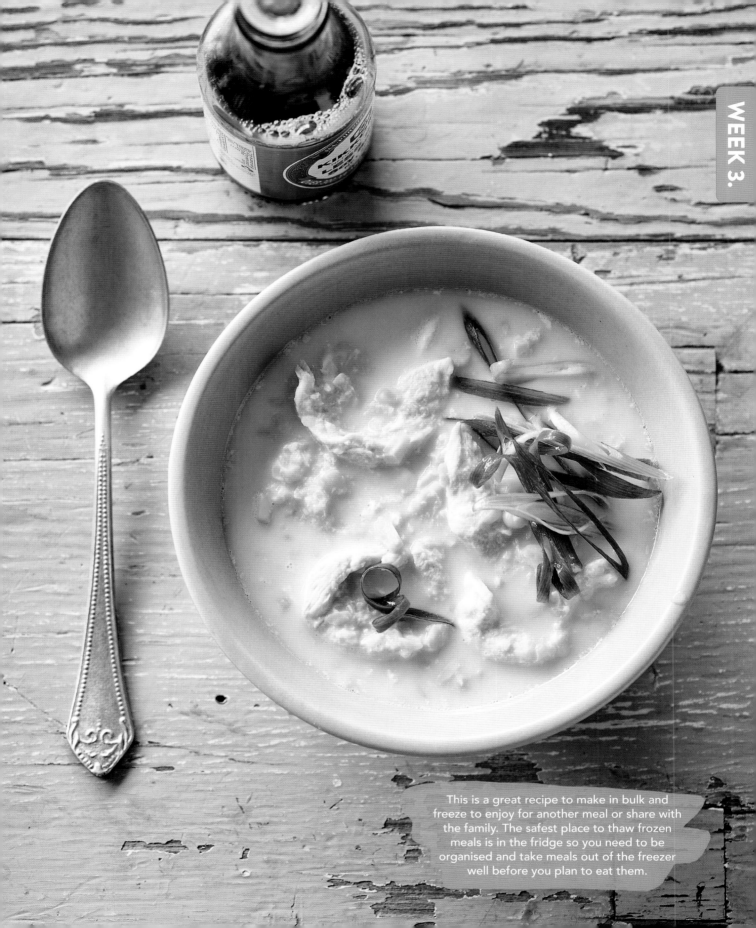

This is a great recipe to make in bulk and freeze to enjoy for another meal or share with the family. The safest place to thaw frozen meals is in the fridge so you need to be organised and take meals out of the freezer well before you plan to eat them.

TUNA AND CITRUS SALAD

SERVES: 2 **PREPARATION TIME:** 10 MINUTES

2 tablespoons reduced-fat
  Greek-style yoghurt
2 teaspoons extra virgin olive oil
2 teaspoons lime juice
1 garlic clove, crushed
salt and freshly ground black
  pepper
60 g mixed lettuce leaves
2 radishes, sliced
½ medium orange, peeled and
  cut into slices
½ medium grapefruit, peeled
  and cut into slices
180 g tinned tuna in spring
  water, drained
2 tablespoons dried cranberries

Combine the yoghurt, olive oil, lime juice and garlic in a small bowl and whisk to combine. Season with salt and pepper.

Arrange the lettuce, radish, orange and grapefruit in two bowls and top with the tuna. Drizzle over the dressing, then sprinkle with cranberries and serve.

NUTRI DETAILS PER SERVE

289 cals/1201 kjs
Protein: 29.5 g
Fibre: 6 g
Total fat: 8 g
Sat fat: 2 g
Carbs: 20.5 g
Total sugar: 19 g
Free sugar: 0.0 g

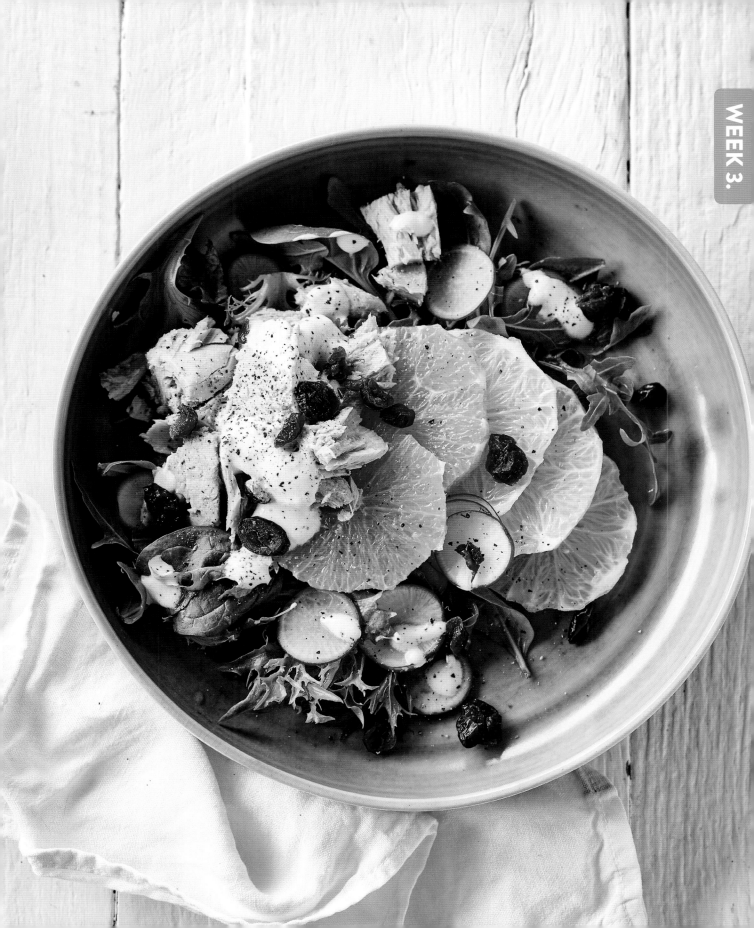

When looking at the recipes from your weekly meal plans, see what you can make in advance on 'meal prep' day to make your busy life easier. For example, you could pre-cook the pasta and chicken and hard-boil the eggs for this recipe. Allow to cool, then store in airtight containers in the fridge for up to 2–3 days so you can quickly assemble this healthy salad when you are ready for it.

CHICKEN PASTA CAESAR SALAD

SERVES: 2   PREPARATION TIME: 15 MINUTES   COOKING TIME: 10 MINUTES

80 g wholemeal pasta (any shape)

cooking oil spray

100 g chicken breast fillet

salt and freshly ground black pepper

60 g cos lettuce leaves, roughly chopped

1 celery stalk, diced

2 slices lean smoked ham, chopped

1 hard-boiled free-range egg, peeled and sliced

1 slice wholegrain or gluten-free bread of choice

2 tablespoons reduced-fat Greek-style yoghurt

1 teaspoon Dijon mustard

2 tablespoons lemon juice

2 tablespoons shredded parmesan

Cook the pasta in a saucepan of boiling water until al dente. Drain.

Meanwhile, lightly spray a frying pan with cooking oil spray and place over medium–high heat. Season the chicken with salt and pepper, then add to the pan and cook for 4–5 minutes each side or until cooked through. Allow to cool, then slice.

Combine the lettuce and celery in a serving bowl, then toss through the cooked pasta. Add the chicken, ham and egg and gently toss again.

Toast the bread and cut it into cubes, then scatter over the salad.

Combine the yoghurt, mustard and lemon juice in a small bowl and whisk to combine. Season with salt and pepper. Drizzle the dressing over the salad and toss well.

Divide the salad between two bowls, sprinkle with parmesan and serve.

NUTRI DETAILS PER SERVE

368 cals/1549 kjs
Protein: 33.8 g
Fibre: 5.7 g
Total fat: 10.6 g
Sat fat: 3.9 g
Carbs: 30.7 g
Total sugar: 3 g
Free sugar: 0.0 g

CRUSTLESS QUICHES

SERVES: 2 **PREPARATION TIME:** 10 MINUTES **COOKING TIME:** 20 MINUTES

cooking oil spray
½ small zucchini, grated
1 medium carrot, grated
3 tablespoons grated reduced-fat cheddar
4 free-range eggs
2 tablespoons reduced-fat milk of choice
½ teaspoon dried Italian herbs
mixed salad leaves, to serve
2 tablespoons tomato passata

Preheat the oven to 200°C. Lightly spray six holes of a standard muffin tray with cooking oil spray and line with baking paper or patty pan cases.

Place the zucchini, carrot, cheese, eggs, milk and herbs in a bowl and mix to combine.

Spoon the batter evenly into the muffin holes and bake for 15–20 minutes or until firm on top and cooked through.

Place three quiches on each plate and serve with mixed salad leaves and tomato passata for dipping.

NUTRI DETAILS PER SERVE

277 cals/1160 kjs
Protein: 23.7 g
Fibre: 3.7 g
Total fat: 16.8 g
Sat fat: 7.3 g
Carbs: 5.9 g
Total sugar: 4.9 g
Free sugar: 0.0 g

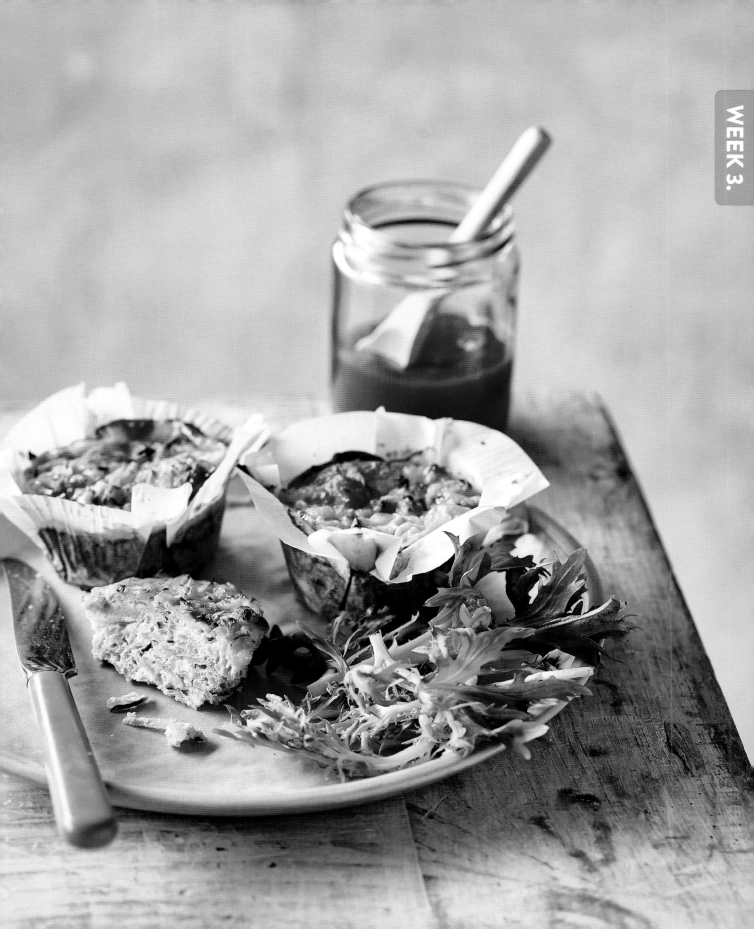

GREEN MAC AND CHEESE

SERVES: 2   **PREPARATION TIME:** 5 MINUTES   **COOKING TIME:** 25 MINUTES

½ cup macaroni
1 cup reduced-fat milk of choice
2 teaspoons cornflour
60 g kale leaves, shredded
½ cup grated reduced-fat cheddar
salt and freshly ground black pepper

NUTRI DETAILS PER SERVE

318 cals/1335 kjs
Protein: 25 g
Fibre: 6 g
Total fat: 5 g
Sat fat: 1.5 g
Carbs: 40 g
Total sugar: 9 g
Free sugar: 0.0 g

Preheat the oven to 180°C.

Cook the macaroni in a saucepan of boiling water for 8–10 minutes or until al dente. Drain.

Meanwhile, pour the milk into a saucepan and gently heat to just below boiling point. Blend the cornflour with 2 tablespoons water and stir into the hot milk, stirring constantly until the mixture thickens. Add the kale and cheese and stir until the cheese has melted into the sauce, then stir through the drained macaroni. Season with salt and pepper.

Pour the mixture into a 1 litre baking dish and bake for 15 minutes or until the top is golden and everything is heated through.

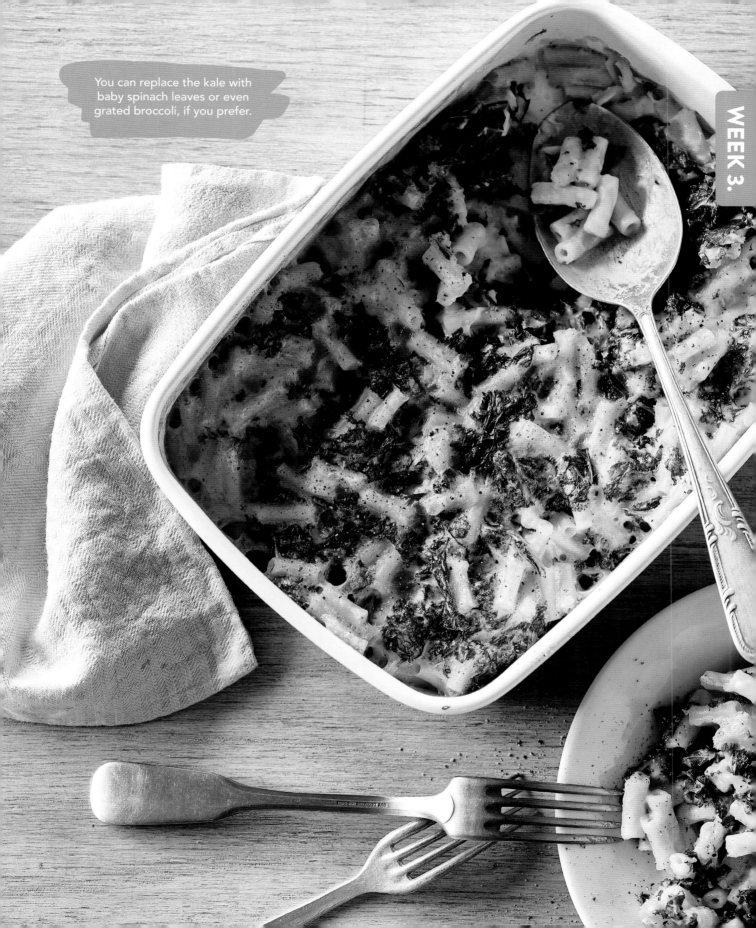

You can replace the kale with baby spinach leaves or even grated broccoli, if you prefer.

MARINATED SALMON WITH QUINOA AND ROAST VEGETABLE SALAD

SERVES: 4   PREPARATION TIME: 15 MINUTES, PLUS MARINATING TIME
COOKING TIME: 40 MINUTES

- 2 tablespoons salt-reduced soy sauce
- 1 tablespoon minced ginger
- 2 tablespoons finely grated lemon zest
- 400 g salmon fillet (or firm fish of choice), skin and bones removed
- 2 small zucchini, chopped
- 1 red capsicum, seeds removed, chopped
- ½ red onion, roughly chopped
- 1 cup quinoa, rinsed
- 60 g baby spinach leaves
- ⅓ cup lemon juice
- ⅓ cup mint leaves
- 1 teaspoon dried chilli flakes

NUTRI DETAILS PER SERVE

416 cals/1739 kjs
Protein: 29.1 g
Fibre: 6 g
Total fat: 16.6 g
Sat fat: 4 g
Carbs: 33.8 g
Total sugar: 9 g
Free sugar: 0.0 g

Combine the soy sauce, ginger and lemon zest in a glass or ceramic dish. Add the salmon and turn to coat, then place in the fridge to marinate for 1 hour.

Preheat the oven to 180°C and line two baking trays with baking paper.

Spread out the zucchini, capsicum and onion on one of the prepared trays and roast for 25 minutes or until tender.

While the vegetables are cooking, place the quinoa and 2 cups water in a saucepan and bring to the boil. Reduce the heat and simmer, covered, for 15 minutes or until tender and most of the liquid has been absorbed. Fluff up with a fork.

Meanwhile, remove the salmon from the dish and pat with paper towel to remove any excess marinade.

Heat a non-stick frying pan over medium–high heat, add the salmon and cook for 1–2 minutes each side. Transfer to the second lined tray and bake for 7–10 minutes or until cooked to your liking.

Toss the roast vegetables and quinoa together in a large bowl, then add the spinach, lemon juice, mint and chilli flakes and toss again to combine.

Divide the salad among four plates. Roughly flake the salmon and arrange on top to serve.

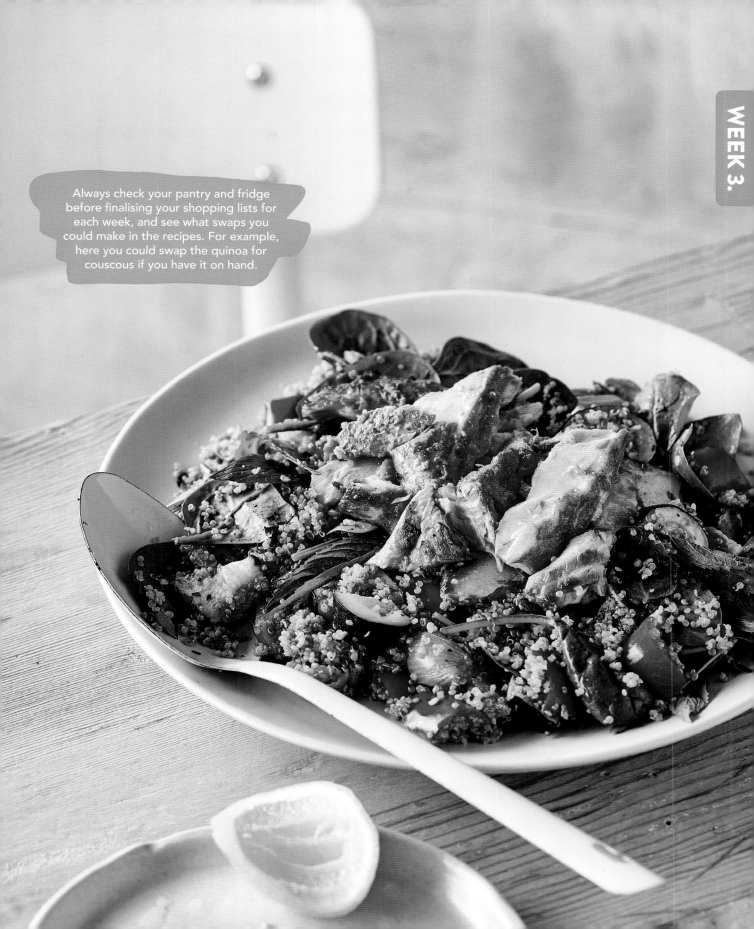

Always check your pantry and fridge before finalising your shopping lists for each week, and see what swaps you could make in the recipes. For example, here you could swap the quinoa for couscous if you have it on hand.

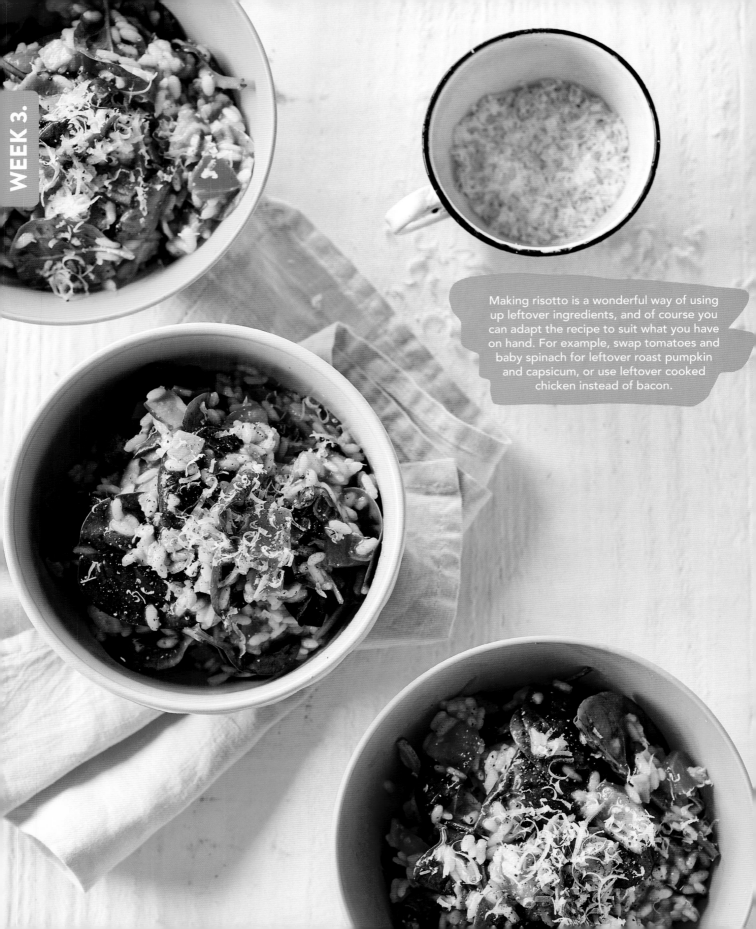

Making risotto is a wonderful way of using up leftover ingredients, and of course you can adapt the recipe to suit what you have on hand. For example, swap tomatoes and baby spinach for leftover roast pumpkin and capsicum, or use leftover cooked chicken instead of bacon.

BACON, SPINACH AND TOMATO RISOTTO

SERVES: 4   PREPARATION TIME: 5 MINUTES   COOKING TIME: 35 MINUTES

1 tablespoon extra-virgin olive oil

6 lean bacon rashers, trimmed and diced

1 cup arborio rice

3 cups salt-reduced hot vegetable stock, plus extra if needed

2 tomatoes, diced

120 g baby spinach leaves

salt and freshly ground black pepper

⅓ cup grated parmesan

Heat the olive oil in a large heavy-based saucepan over medium–high heat. Add the bacon and cook for 4–5 minutes or until crispy. Add the rice and stir for a few minutes to coat the grains in the oil.

Add the stock, 3 tablespoons at a time, stirring until each addition has been absorbed by the rice before adding the next. This will take approximately 20 minutes.

Add the tomato and spinach with the last addition of stock, then cover with a lid and reduce to a gentle simmer for 10 minutes or until the rice is cooked through and tender (add a little more stock if needed).

Season to taste with salt and pepper and sprinkle with parmesan to serve.

NUTRI DETAILS PER SERVE

338 cals/1421 kjs
Protein: 16 g
Fibre: 1.9 g
Total fat: 10.7 g
Sat fat: 3.5 g
Carbs: 43.3 g
Total sugar: 1.7 g
Free sugar: 0.0 g

TANDOORI LAMB WITH COUSCOUS SALAD

SERVES: 4   PREPARATION TIME: 15 MINUTES   COOKING TIME: 10 MINUTES

1 cup couscous

1 cup boiling water

salt and freshly ground black pepper

2 tablespoons tandoori paste

⅓ cup reduced-fat Greek-style yoghurt

8 (about 480 g) lean lamb cutlets, excess fat trimmed

1 Lebanese cucumber, chopped

4 spring onions, finely sliced

⅓ cup chopped mint leaves

2 tomatoes, chopped

3 tablespoons lemon juice

1 tablespoon extra-virgin olive oil

Place the couscous in a heatproof bowl and cover with the boiling water. Cover the bowl with plastic wrap and set aside for 5 minutes. When all the liquid has been absorbed by the couscous, fluff it up with a fork and season with salt and pepper.

Mix together the tandoori paste and yoghurt and spread over the lamb. Set aside to marinate for 5 minutes.

Meanwhile, place the couscous, cucumber, spring onion, mint, tomato and lemon juice in a bowl and toss to combine. Season with salt and pepper.

Heat the olive oil in a large frying pan over medium heat. Add the lamb and cook for 4 minutes each side or until cooked to your liking.

Serve the tandoori lamb with the couscous salad on the side.

NUTRI DETAILS PER SERVE

449 cals/1885 kjs
Protein: 39.1 g
Fibre: 2.4 g
Total fat: 18.4 g
Sat fat: 4.9 g
Carbs: 30 g
Total sugar: 3.6 g
Free sugar: 0.0 g

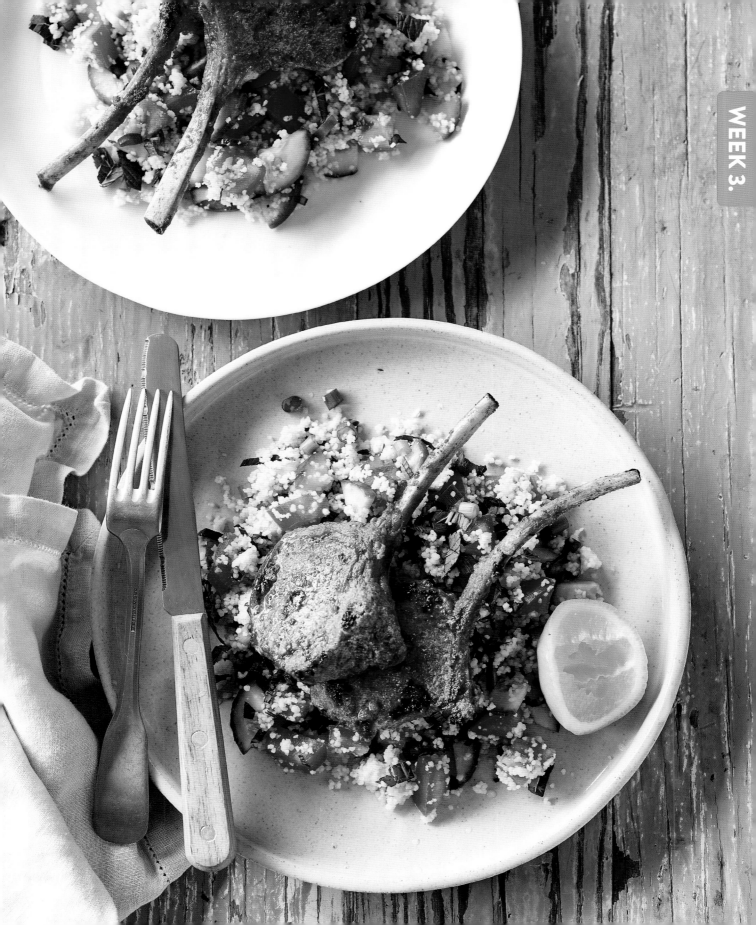

QUICK CHICKEN LAKSA

SERVES: 4   **PREPARATION TIME:** 10 MINUTES   **COOKING TIME:** 15 MINUTES

cooking oil spray

⅓ cup laksa paste (store-bought is fine)

1.25 litres salt-reduced chicken stock

600 g chicken breast fillets, cut into thick strips

120 ml coconut cream

4 small heads bok choy, trimmed and chopped

Lightly spray a large saucepan with cooking oil spray and place over medium–high heat. Add the laksa paste and cook for 1 minute or until fragrant, then add the stock and bring to the boil.

Add the chicken and simmer for 5 minutes or until cooked through. Add the coconut cream and bok choy and simmer for a few more minutes or until the bok choy is tender.

Ladle the laksa into four bowls and serve.

NUTRI DETAILS PER SERVE

390 cals/1636 kjs
Protein: 38 g
Fibre: 4 g
Total fat: 23 g
Sat fat: 9 g
Carbs: 6 g
Total sugar: 9 g
Free sugar: 3 g

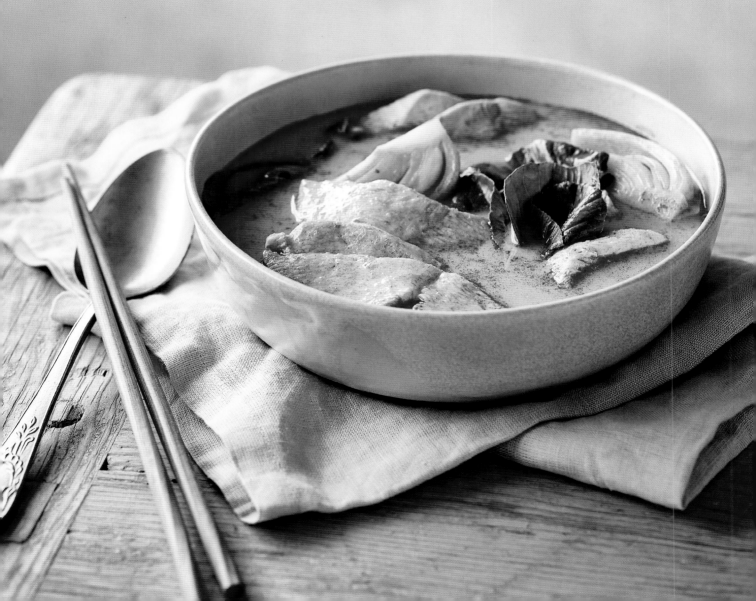

GREEK BEEF BURGERS

SERVES: 4   PREPARATION TIME: 15 MINUTES   COOKING TIME: 10 MINUTES

320 g lean beef mince
⅓ cup finely chopped mint leaves
1 teaspoon dried oregano
½ brown onion, grated
⅓ cup green olives, chopped
80 g reduced-fat feta, crumbled
cooking oil spray
4 wholegrain rolls
60 g mixed lettuce leaves
1 Lebanese cucumber, cut into long ribbons or sliced
2 tomatoes, sliced

Combine the mince, mint, oregano, onion, olives and feta in a bowl. Divide into four even portions and shape into patties. Refrigerate for 20 minutes.

Lightly spray a large non-stick frying pan with cooking oil spray and place over medium–high heat. Add the patties and cook for 3–4 minutes each side or until cooked through.

Cut the rolls in half and top the bases with the lettuce, cucumber and tomato. Add one patty to each, then sandwich with the remaining roll halves and serve.

NUTRI DETAILS PER SERVE

405 cals/1702 kjs
Protein: 33 g
Fibre: 6.9 g
Total fat: 14.2 g
Sat fat: 5.4 g
Carbs: 32.8 g
Total sugar: 5.9 g
Free sugar: 0.0 g

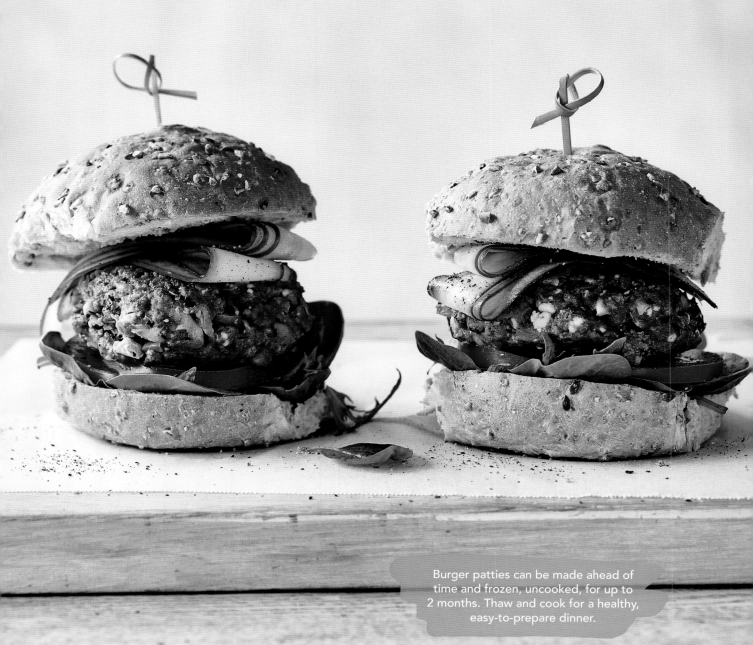

Burger patties can be made ahead of time and frozen, uncooked, for up to 2 months. Thaw and cook for a healthy, easy-to-prepare dinner.

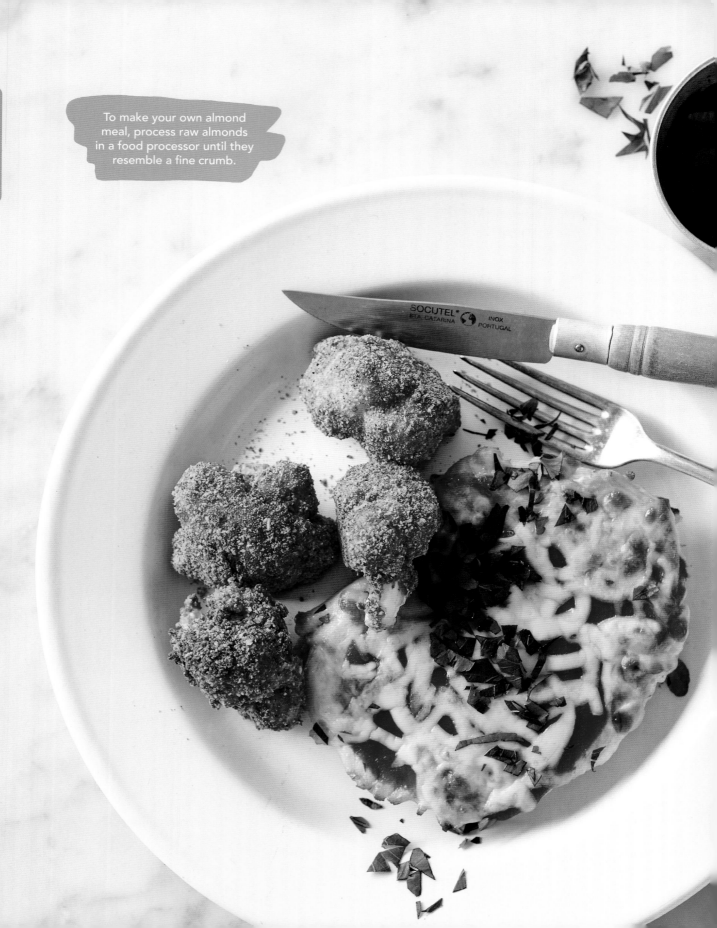

To make your own almond meal, process raw almonds in a food processor until they resemble a fine crumb.

NAKED CHICKEN PARMA WITH POPCORN CAULIFLOWER

SERVES: 4   PREPARATION TIME: 15 MINUTES   COOKING TIME: 30 MINUTES

50 g almond meal

1 teaspoon chilli powder

1 teaspoon smoked paprika

1 teaspoon ground cumin

1 teaspoon ground turmeric

salt and freshly ground black pepper

1 cup reduced-fat milk of choice

1 cup plain wholemeal flour

400 g cauliflower, cut into florets

2 × 200 g chicken breast fillets, halved horizontally

⅓ cup tomato passata

⅓ cup grated reduced-fat mozzarella

2 tablespoons chopped flat-leaf parsley, to serve

NUTRI DETAILS PER SERVE

396 cals/1664 kjs
Protein: 35.4 g
Fibre: 7.3 g
Total fat: 7.3 g
Sat fat: 3.7 g
Carbs: 28.7g
Total sugar: 7.2 g
Free sugar: 0.0 g

Preheat the oven to 180°C and line two baking trays with baking paper.

Combine the almond meal, spices and salt and pepper in a bowl to make a crumb.

In another bowl, mix together the milk and wholemeal flour to make a batter.

Coat the cauliflower florets in the batter, then toss in the spiced crumb mixture. Arrange the cauliflower on one of the prepared trays and bake for 25–30 minutes or until golden brown and crisp.

Meanwhile, place the chicken breasts on a chopping board, cover with plastic wrap and lightly tenderise with a mallet or the end of a rolling pin.

Place the chicken on the second lined tray and bake for 15 minutes or until almost cooked. Remove the tray and top the chicken with the passata and cheese, then return to the oven and bake for a further 5 minutes or until the chicken is cooked through and the cheese has melted.

Serve the chicken parma alongside the popcorn cauliflower. Sprinkle with parsley to serve.

LENTIL AND QUINOA SALAD WITH EGGS AND PESTO

SERVES: 4   PREPARATION TIME: 15 MINUTES   COOKING TIME: 15 MINUTES

1 cup quinoa, rinsed

80 g tinned brown lentils, drained and rinsed

1 tablespoon cumin seeds, roasted

2 tomatoes, chopped

⅔ cup chopped flat-leaf parsley leaves

⅔ cup chopped mint leaves

⅓ cup lemon juice

2 tablespoons extra virgin olive oil, plus extra if needed

salt and freshly ground black pepper

2 garlic cloves, crushed

⅔ cup chopped basil leaves

⅓ cup grated parmesan

4 hard-boiled free-range eggs, peeled and sliced

Place the quinoa and 2 cups water in a saucepan and bring to the boil. Reduce the heat and simmer, covered, for 15 minutes or until tender and most of the liquid has been absorbed. Fluff up with a fork.

Combine the quinoa, lentils, cumin seeds, tomato, parsley and mint in a bowl. Drizzle with the lemon juice and 1 tablespoon of the olive oil, and toss to combine. Season with salt and pepper.

Place the garlic and basil in a food processor and process until finely chopped. Add the parmesan and remaining olive oil and process until smooth. Add a little extra oil or some water to loosen if needed.

Divide the quinoa salad among four bowls and arrange the hard-boiled eggs on top.

Dollop over the pesto and serve.

NUTRI DETAILS PER SERVE

407 cals/1704 kjs
Protein: 20.2 g
Fibre: 6.9 g
Total fat: 20.3 g
Sat fat: 5.1 g
Carbs: 32.3 g
Total sugar: 4.3 g
Free sugar: 0.0 g

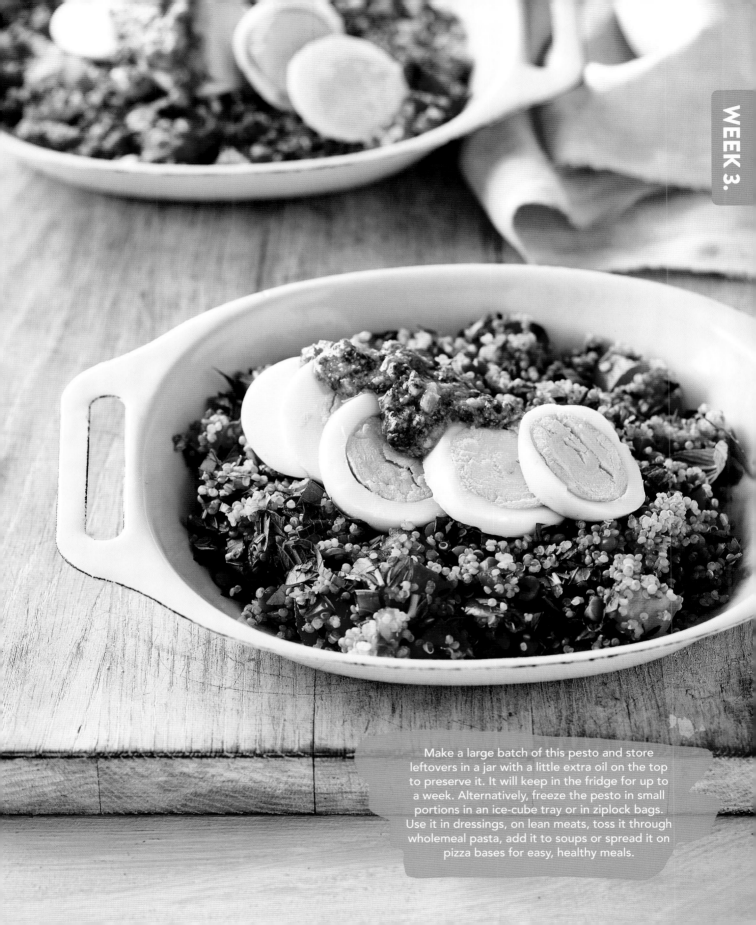

Make a large batch of this pesto and store leftovers in a jar with a little extra oil on the top to preserve it. It will keep in the fridge for up to a week. Alternatively, freeze the pesto in small portions in an ice-cube tray or in ziplock bags. Use it in dressings, on lean meats, toss it through wholemeal pasta, add it to soups or spread it on pizza bases for easy, healthy meals.

SESAME AND SWEET POTATO DIP

SERVES: 4   **PREPARATION TIME:** 5 MINUTES, PLUS SOAKING TIME   **COOKING TIME:** 10 MINUTES

40 g unsalted cashews

1 small sweet potato, peeled and chopped

2 tablespoons tahini

1 tablespoon chopped chives, plus extra to garnish

salt and freshly ground black pepper

24 plain rice crackers

Soak the cashews in water overnight. Drain when you are ready to prepare the dip.

Steam the sweet potato until tender. Set aside to cool.

Place the soaked cashews, sweet potato, tahini and chives in a blender and blitz until smooth. Season with salt and pepper and garnish with the extra chives.

Divide the dip into four portions and serve each portion with six rice crackers. Any leftover dip will keep in an airtight container in the fridge for 3–4 days.

NUTRI DETAILS PER SERVE

148 cals/621 kjs
Protein: 4 g
Fibre: 3 g
Total fat: 9.1 g
Sat fat: 1.5 g
Carbs: 14.5 g
Total sugar: 3.7 g
Free sugar: 0.0 g

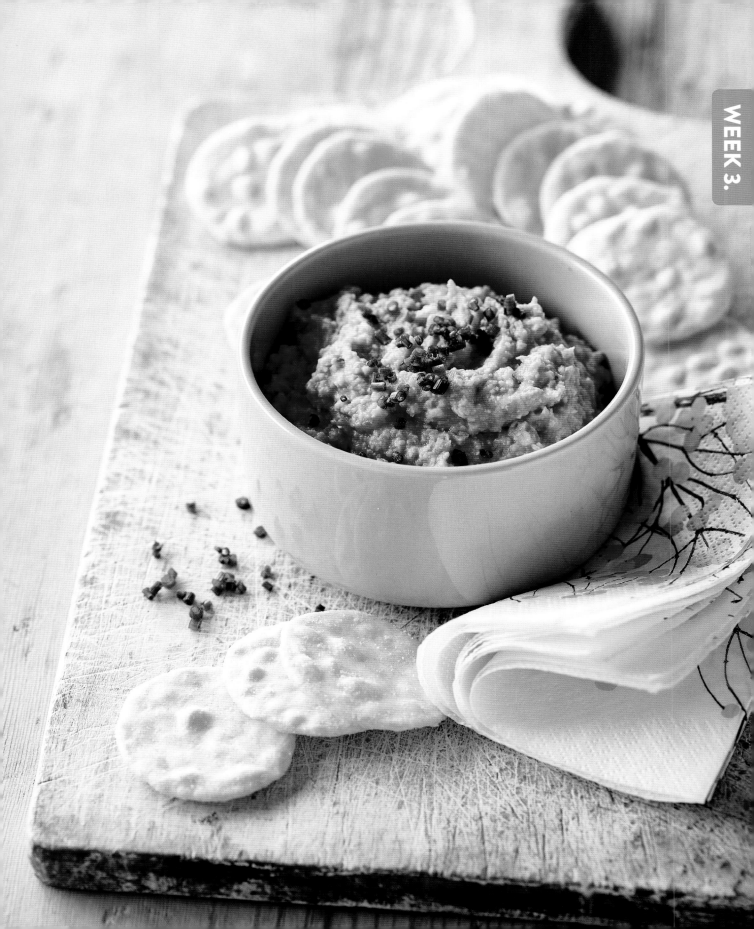

SPINACH BALLS

SERVES: 4   **PREPARATION TIME:** 15 MINUTES   **COOKING TIME:** 25 MINUTES

---

280 g frozen spinach, thawed
2 teaspoons coconut oil
1 brown onion, finely chopped
1 ¼ cups dried wholemeal breadcrumbs
2 ½ teaspoons dried Italian herbs
3 free-range eggs
2 tablespoons grated parmesan
salt and freshly ground black pepper
lemon wedges, to serve (optional)

NUTRI DETAILS PER SERVE

267 cals/1120 kjs
Protein: 15 g
Fibre: 5 g
Total fat: 10 g
Sat fat: 5 g
Carbs: 27 g
Total sugar: 3 g
Free sugar: 0.0 g

Preheat the oven to 180°C and line a baking tray with baking paper.

Squeeze the excess water from the spinach, then roughly chop.

Melt the coconut oil in a small frying pan over medium heat. Add the onion and cook until softened.

Transfer the onion to a bowl, then add the spinach, breadcrumbs, herbs, eggs and parmesan and mix until well combined. Season with salt and pepper.

Roll the mixture into 20 bite-sized balls. Place on the prepared tray and bake for 20 minutes or until golden and cooked through. Serve five balls per serve with a wedge of lemon, if desired.

Any leftovers will keep in an airtight container in the fridge for 3 days or in the freezer for up to 3 months. Thaw and reheat as required.

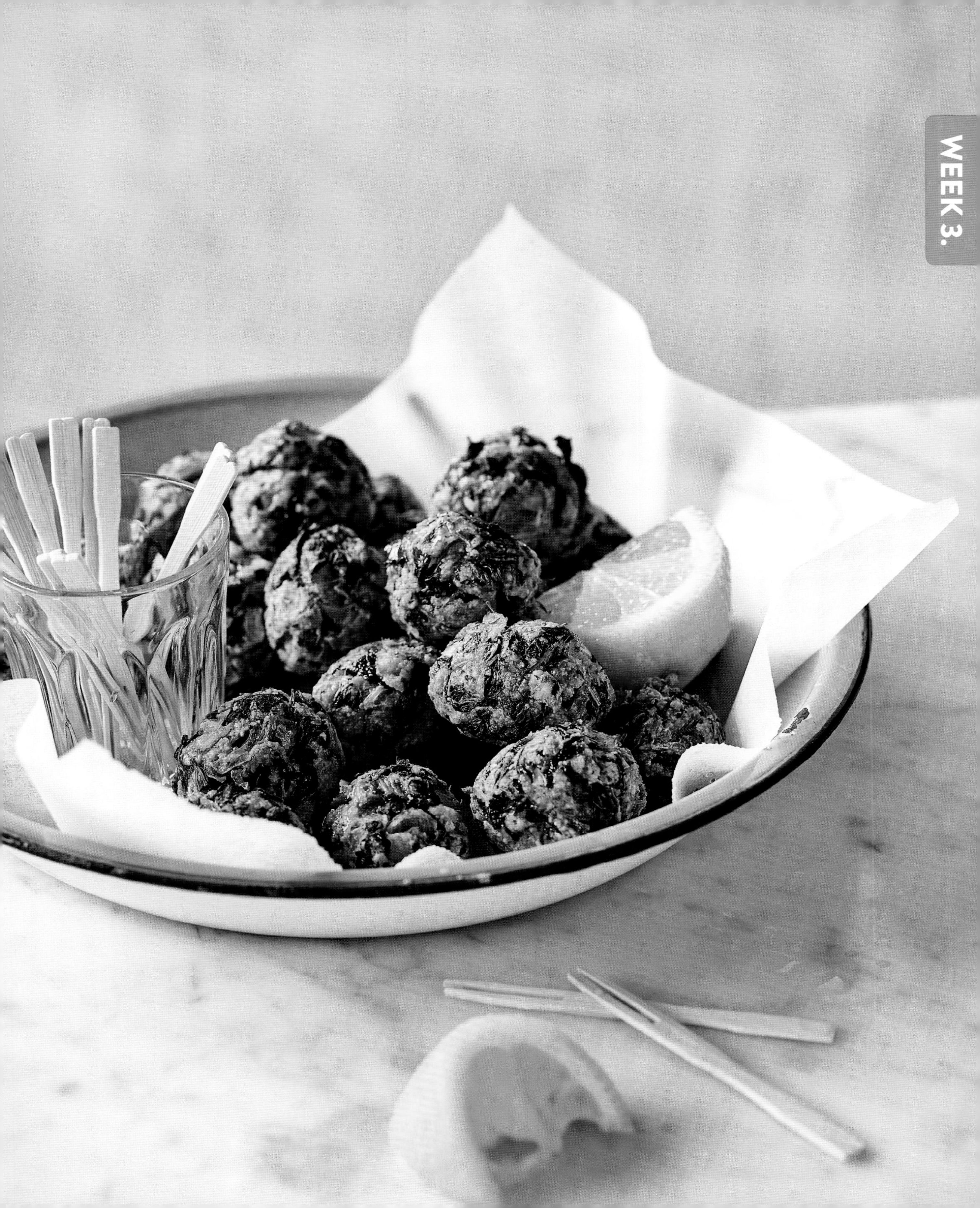

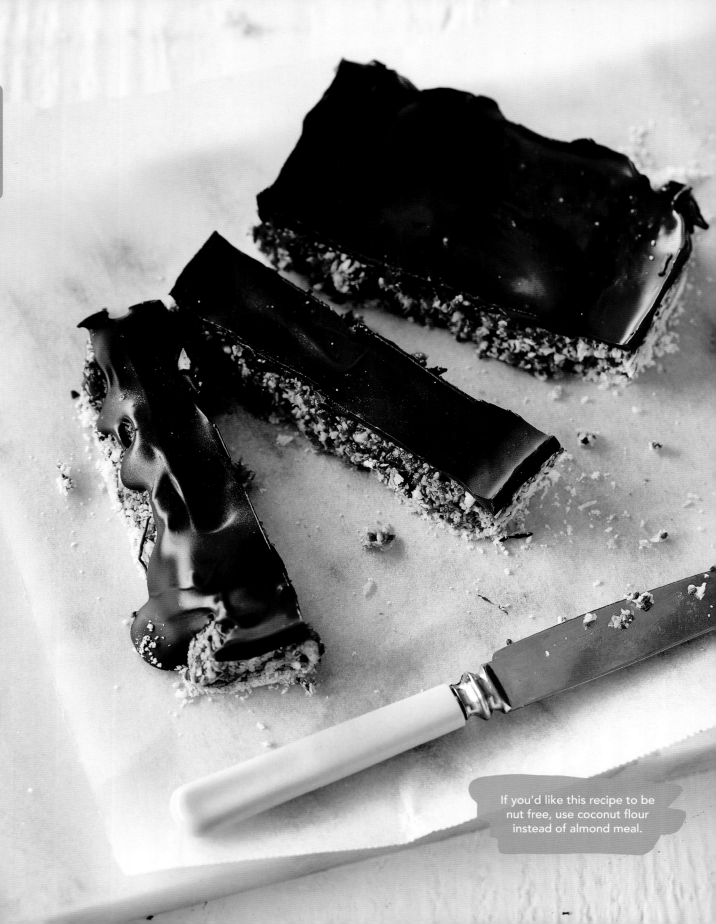

If you'd like this recipe to be nut free, use coconut flour instead of almond meal.

CHERRY-CHOC SLICE

SERVES: 5   **PREPARATION TIME:** 10 MINUTES, PLUS CHILLING TIME   **COOKING TIME:** 5 MINUTES

150 g fresh or frozen cherries, thawed and drained if frozen, pitted

2 ½ tablespoons coconut oil

½ cup desiccated coconut

2 tablespoons chia seeds

60 g dark chocolate (70% cocoa solids)

1 tablespoon almond meal

NUTRI DETAILS PER SERVE

253 cals/1062 kjs
Protein: 2.6 g
Fibre: 4.2 g
Total fat: 21.3 g
Sat fat: 17.5 g
Carbs: 13.3 g
Total sugar: 10.3 g
Free sugar: 6.6 g

Place the cherries, coconut oil, coconut and chia seeds in a food processor and process until well combined. It doesn't have to be completely smooth – some small lumps of cherry are fine and add to the texture of the slice.

Line a loaf tin with baking paper. Spoon the mixture into the tin and smooth the surface. Place the tin in the fridge while you melt the chocolate.

Break the chocolate into small pieces and melt in a small heatproof bowl set over a saucepan of simmering water, stirring occasionally.

Pour the melted chocolate over the cherry mixture and tilt the tin to ensure a thin, even coating of chocolate. Return the tin to the fridge for at least 4 hours.

When the slice is set, dust a chopping board liberally with the almond meal, and place the slice on the board. This will give it a slightly cakey base. Using a hot knife, cut the slice into five even pieces.

Store any leftovers in an airtight container in the fridge for up to 2 weeks or in the freezer for up to 3 months.

PAPRIKA PARMESAN CHIPS

SERVES: 4   **PREPARATION TIME:** 5 MINUTES   **COOKING TIME:** 10 MINUTES

4 wholemeal tortillas
⅓ cup grated parmesan
1 teaspoon smoked paprika
⅓ cup reduced-fat Greek-style
  yoghurt
⅔ cup tomato salsa
  (store-bought is fine)

NUTRI DETAILS PER SERVE

115 cals/481 kjs
Protein: 5.5 g
Fibre: 1.6 g
Total fat: 4 g
Sat fat: 2.3 g
Carbs: 12.9 g
Total sugar: 4.2 g
Free sugar: 0.0 g

Preheat the oven to 180°C and line a baking tray with baking paper.

Cut the tortillas into triangles and place in a single layer on the prepared tray. Bake for 5 minutes. Turn the chips over, sprinkle with the parmesan and paprika and bake for a further 3–5 minutes or until crisp and golden.

Divide the chips into four equal portions. Serve each portion with 1 tablespoon yoghurt and 2 tablespoons salsa.

Store any leftover chips in an airtight container in the pantry for 4–5 days.

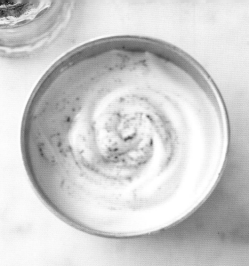

These chips are great to make when you're entertaining. You can also use wholemeal pita breads and serve them with your favourite dips.

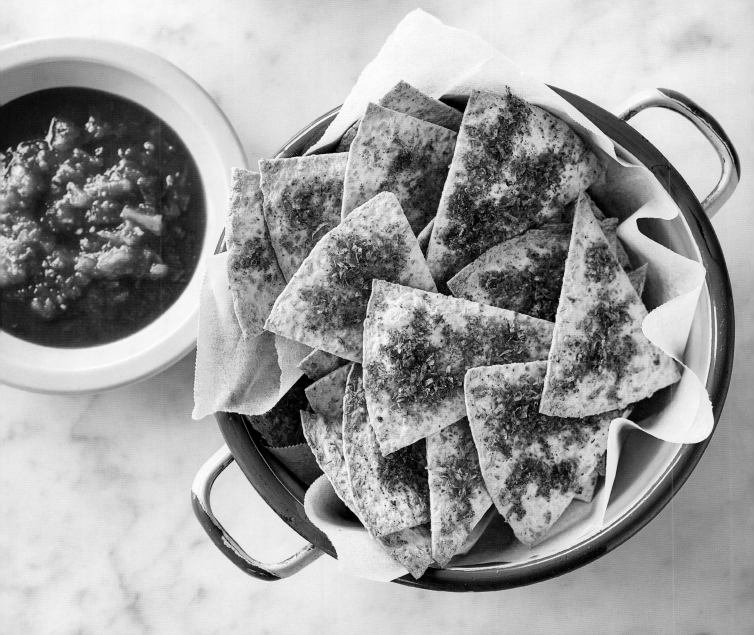

BLUEBERRY MOUSSE WITH PISTACHIOS

SERVES: 4   **PREPARATION TIME:** 10 MINUTES

100 g silken tofu

2 tablespoons almond meal

1 cup blueberries (fresh or frozen)

1 tablespoon chia seeds

1 tablespoon desiccated coconut

1 teaspoon vanilla extract

1 tablespoon pure maple syrup

⅓ cup reduced-fat milk of choice

1 tablespoon coconut oil, melted

2 teaspoons unsalted pistachios, chopped

Place the tofu, almond meal, blueberries, chia seeds, desiccated coconut, vanilla, maple syrup, milk and coconut oil in a blender and blend until smooth.

Divide the mixture among four serving jars or small glasses (⅓ cup capacity), sprinkle with the chopped pistachios and serve.

Any leftovers may be covered and stored in the fridge for 4–5 days.

NUTRI DETAILS PER SERVE

187 cals/782 kjs
Protein: 4.6 g
Fibre: 3.9 g
Total fat: 13.8 g
Sat fat: 5.7 g
Carbs: 9.1 g
Total sugar: 8.2 g
Free sugar: 3.9 g

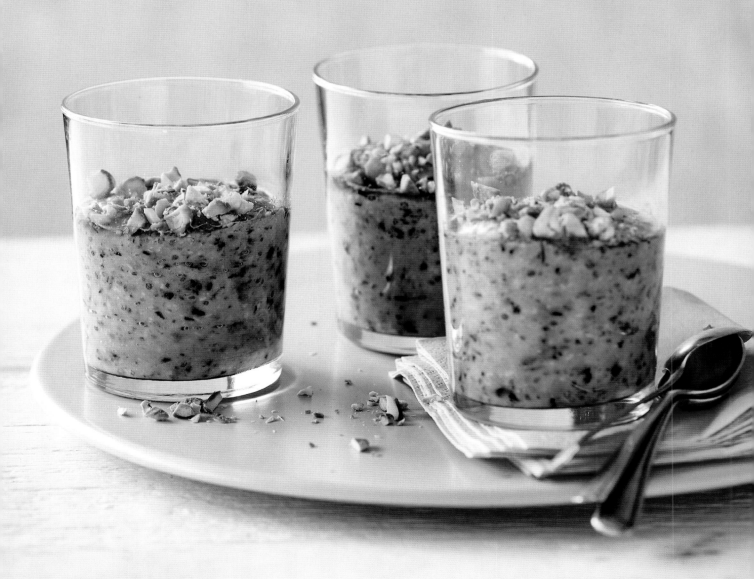

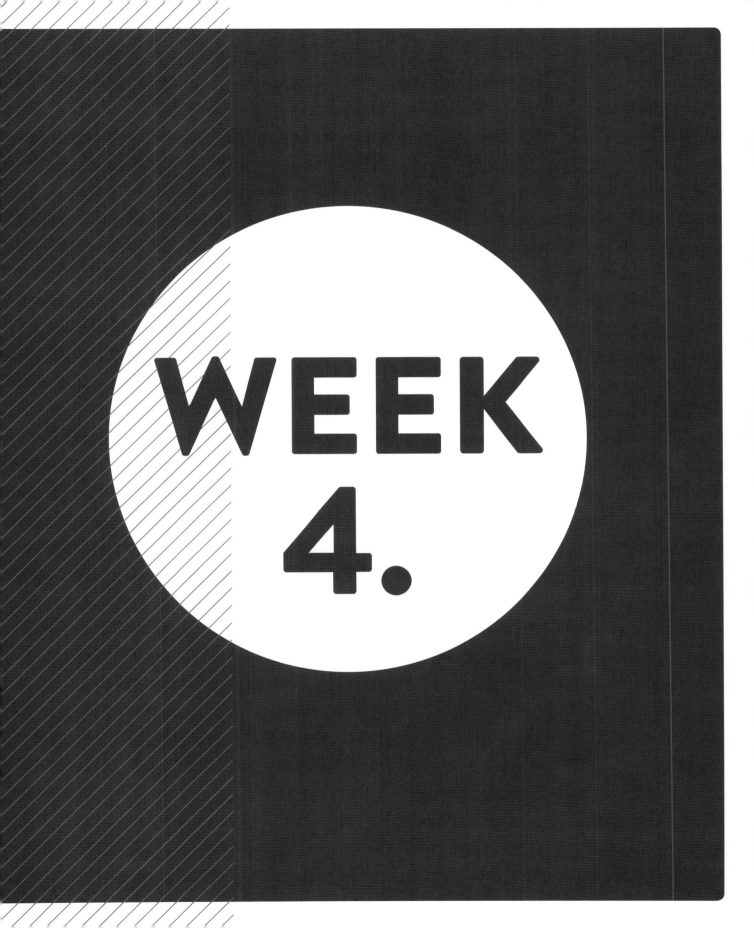

MEAL & EXERCISE PLAN

4.

	MONDAY	TUESDAY	WEDNESDAY
BREAKFAST	Date and Oat Breakfast Slice **p.204** 333 cals	Warm Vanilla and Apple Bircher **p.207** 337 cals	Mushroom Omelette Rolls **p.208** 335 cals
MORNING SNACK	Chocolate Peanut Butter Crumble Balls **p.246** 154 cals	1 orange served with 1 cup herbal tea 54 cals	Raspberry Muffins **p.249** 231 cals
LUNCH	Carrot and Beetroot Slaw with Haloumi **p.218** 336 cals	Thick and Creamy Lentil and Tomato Soup **p.220** 312 cals	Healthy Egg Sandwiches **p.223** 345 cals
EXERCISE	20 minute Metabolic Booster**, Workout 2 (see page 285)	20 minute Body Strong Pilates, Workout 2 (see page 288)	20 minute Deep Core Conditioning*, Workout 2 (see page 291)
AFTERNOON SNACK	1 orange served with 1 cup herbal tea 54 cals	Raspberry Muffins **p.249** 231 cals	Layered Yoghurt and Raspberry Sorbet **p.252** 83 cals
DINNER	Pork with Tangy Coleslaw **p.232** 295 cals	Spanish Rice with Chorizo **p.234** 409 cals	Spicy Beef and Black Bean Salad **p.236** 308 cals
EVENING SNACK	Raspberry Muffins **p.249** 231 cals	Layered Yoghurt and Raspberry Sorbet **p.252** 83 cals	Chocolate Peanut Butter Crumble Balls **p.246** 154 cals
TOTAL CALORIES	**1403 cals**	**1426 cals**	**1456 cals**

** Choose the low-impact 20 Minute Tummy Tamer workout to complete today if you are still recovering from a C-section, abdominal separation, prolapse, or if you have a weak pelvic floor.

THURSDAY	FRIDAY	SATURDAY	SUNDAY
Crunchy Grilled Banana Wrap **p.210** 345 cals	Veggie Scrambled Eggs on Toast **p.212** 345 cals	Mexican Breakfast Potato **p.215** 260 cals	Banana and Choc-Nut French Toast **p.216** 369 cals
Cheese and Chilli Chips with Herby Yoghurt Dip **p.250** 144 cals	Cheese and Chilli Chips with Herby Yoghurt Dip **p.250** 144 cals	Layered Yoghurt and Raspberry Sorbet **p.252** 83 cals	Cheese and Chilli Chips with Herby Yoghurt Dip **p.250** 144 cals
Lime and Coconut Chicken Rice **p.224** 350 cals	Chilli, Tuna and Avocado Open Sandwich **p.226** 306 cals	Ochazuke **p.228** 362 cals	Pumpkin, Bacon and Sweet Potato Soup **p.231** 269 cals
14 minute Total Body Tabata Workout (see page 296)	**20 minute Butt and Thigh*, Workout 2 (see page 299)**	**20 minute Fat Blaster, Workout 2 (see page 303)**	**Active Recovery Day 2 (see page 305)**
Chocolate Peanut Butter Crumble Balls **p.246** 154 cals	Raspberry Muffins **p.249** 231 cals	Chickpea Fries with Mint Sauce **p.255** 367 cals	Chocolate Peanut Butter Crumble Balls **p.246** 154 cals
Fish with Olive and Chilli Sauce **p.239** 228 cals	Ultimate Bean Nachos **p.240** 415 cals	Thai Calamari Salad **p.242** 286 cals	Satay Fried Rice with Egg **p.244** 433 cals
Raspberry Muffins **p.249** 231 cals	1 orange served with 1 cup herbal tea 54 cals	1 orange served with 1 cup herbal tea 54 cals	Layered Yoghurt and Raspberry Sorbet **p.252** 83 cals
1452 cals	**1495 cals**	**1412 cals**	**1452 cals**

*Choose the low-impact variation of this workout if you are still recovering from a C-section, abdominal separation, prolapse, or if you have a weak pelvic floor.

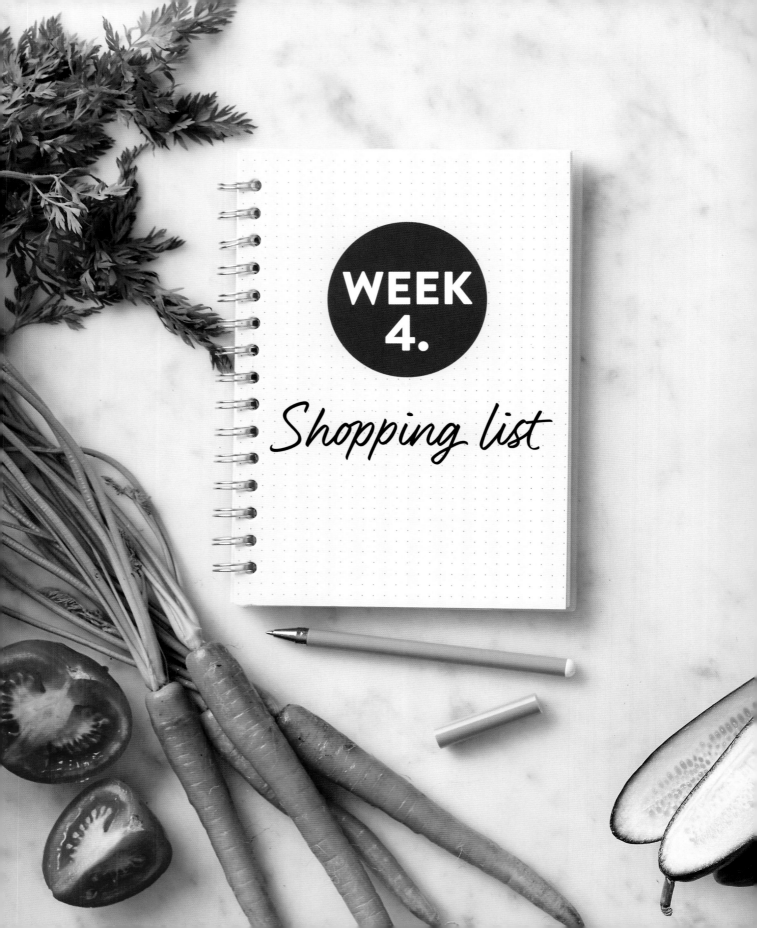

WEEK 4.

Shopping list

Vegetables

Baby spinach leaves 150 g
Beetroot 2
Cabbage, white 200 g
Capsicums, red 3
Carrots 14
Cherry tomatoes 400 g
Chilli, bird's eye 4
Corn kernels 400 g (or used tinned)
Cucumber, Lebanese 2
Fennel ½ bulb
Garlic 3 cloves
Lettuce, cos 60 g
Lettuce, mixed leaves 210 g
Mushrooms, small 115 g
Onions, brown 3
Onion, red 1
Potatoes, medium 2
Pumpkin 450 g
Rocket leaves 150 g
Spring onions 13
Sweet potato, small 1
Tomatoes 11

Fruit

Apples, red 3
Avocados 3
Bananas 4
Lemons 6
Limes 3
Oranges 4
Raspberries 500 g (or use frozen)

Fresh herbs

Basil ½ bunch
Chives ½ bunch
Coriander 2 bunches
Flat-leaf parsley 3 bunches
Mint 1 bunch

Meat, fish, poultry

Bacon rashers, lean and trimmed (2) 55 g
Beef, sirloin steak, lean 320 g
Calamari, fresh or frozen 600 g
Chicken breast fillets 160 g
Chorizo sausages (2) 280 g
Eggs, free range 22
Fish fillets, white 600 g
Pork fillet 600 g

Dairy

Cheddar, reduced-fat grated 80 g
Haloumi 100 g
Yoghurt, reduced-fat natural
   Greek-style 735 g

Breads, grains, cereals and nuts

Bread of choice, wholemeal
   or gluten free, 16 slices
Mountain bread wraps, wholemeal 6

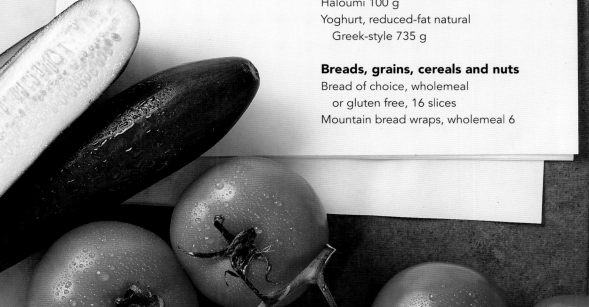

DATE AND OAT BREAKFAST SLICE

SERVES: 6   **PREPARATION TIME:** 5 MINUTES   **COOKING TIME:** 30 MINUTES

2 small apples, grated
3 tablespoons coconut oil
1 cup pitted dates, chopped
1 cup rolled oats
1 cup almond meal
1 teaspoon ground cinnamon

NUTRI DETAILS PER SERVE

333 cals/1398 kjs
Protein: 5.6 g
Fibre: 6.8 g
Total fat: 14.3 g
Sat fat: 8.3 g
Carbs: 50.7 g
Total sugar: 26.3 g
Free sugar: 0.0 g

Combine the apple, coconut oil, dates and ⅓ cup water in a saucepan and bring to the boil.

Reduce the heat and simmer for 5 minutes or until the apple is soft and the mixture has thickened. Set aside to cool completely.

Preheat the oven to 180°C and line a slice tin (about 30 cm × 25 cm) with baking paper.

Mix together the rolled oats, almond meal and cinnamon. Stir into the date mixture, then spoon into the prepared tin and smooth the surface.

Bake for 20 minutes or until firm. Cool completely in the tin, then cut into six pieces.

Store any leftovers in an airtight container in the fridge for 4–5 days.

Having a batch of this healthy slice in the fridge or freezer will save you time in the morning and keep your meals budget friendly.

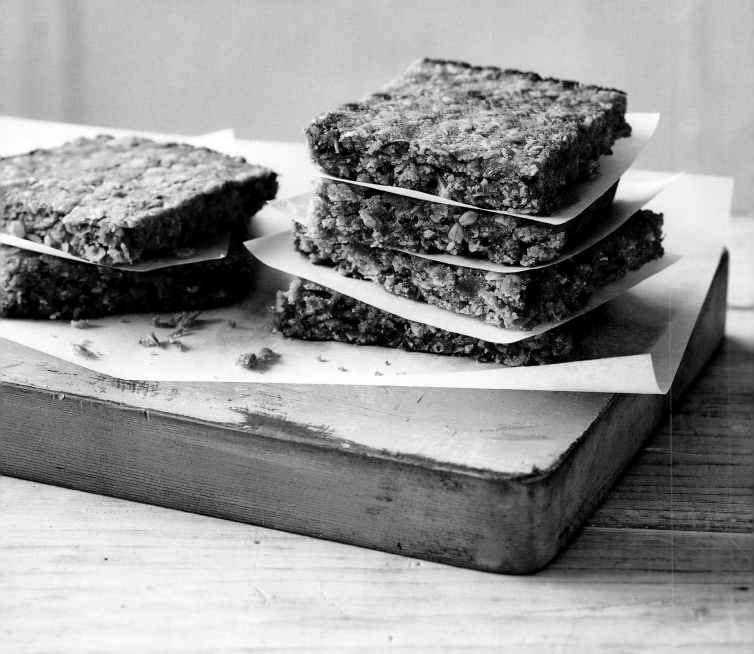

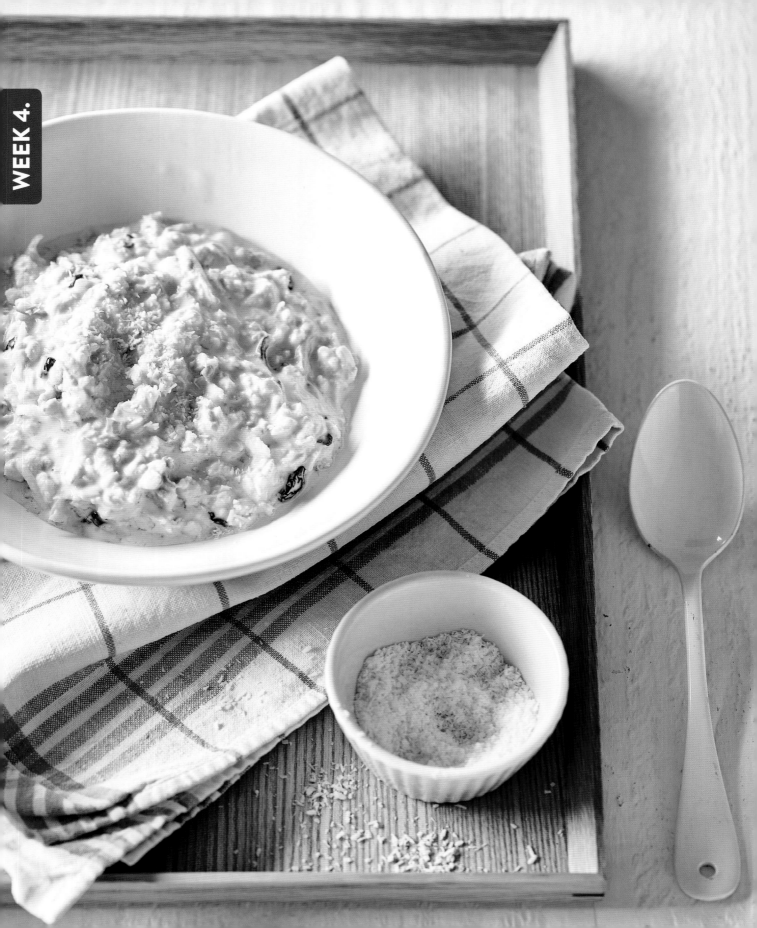

WARM VANILLA AND APPLE BIRCHER

SERVES: 2   **PREPARATION TIME:** 5 MINUTES, PLUS CHILLING TIME   **COOKING TIME:** 5 MINUTES

1 cup rolled oats

½ cup reduced-fat Greek-style yoghurt

1 small apple, grated

2 tablespoons dried cranberries

½ teaspoon vanilla extract

½ cup coconut water

½ cup reduced-fat milk of choice, plus extra to loosen

2 tablespoons desiccated coconut

Combine the oats, yoghurt, apple, cranberries, vanilla, coconut water and milk in a bowl. Cover and refrigerate overnight.

When you are ready to serve, heat the bircher in a saucepan or in the microwave, with a little extra milk to loosen it. It can also be served cold, if desired.

Divide the bircher between two bowls, sprinkle with the desiccated coconut and serve.

NUTRI DETAILS PER SERVE

337 cals/1415 kjs
Protein: 13.7 g
Fibre: 8 g
Total fat: 10.8 g
Sat fat: 6.4 g
Carbs: 42.2 g
Total sugar: 19.9 g
Free sugar: 0.0 g

MUSHROOM OMELETTE ROLLS

SERVES: 2   **PREPARATION TIME:** 10 MINUTES   **COOKING TIME:** 10 MINUTES

4 free-range eggs

1 teaspoon extra virgin olive oil

¼ red onion, finely sliced

75 g mushrooms, sliced

1 medium carrot, cut into matchsticks

2 teaspoons kecap manis (Indonesian sweet soy sauce)

2 slices wholegrain or gluten-free bread of choice

60 g mixed lettuce leaves

2 spring onions, finely sliced

2 teaspoons black or white sesame seeds

Heat a non-stick frying pan over medium–high heat. Lightly beat two eggs, then add them to the pan and swirl to coat the base. Cook for 30 seconds or until just set. Slide the omelette onto a plate and cover to keep warm. Repeat with the remaining eggs to make a second omelette.

Heat the olive oil in the same pan, add the red onion and cook for 2 minutes or until softened. Add the mushroom and carrot and stir-fry for 3 minutes or until tender. Add the kecap manis and stir-fry for 1 minute or until heated through.

Divide the mushroom mixture between the prepared omelettes and roll up tightly to enclose the filling.

Toast the bread and place one slice on each plate with the lettuce. Add the omelette rolls and sprinkle with spring onion and sesame seeds to serve.

NUTRI DETAILS PER SERVE

335 cals/1404 kjs
Protein: 19 g
Fibre: 5 g
Total fat: 18 g
Sat fat: 3.6 g
Carbs: 20.7 g
Total sugar: 4.5 g
Free sugar: 0.0 g

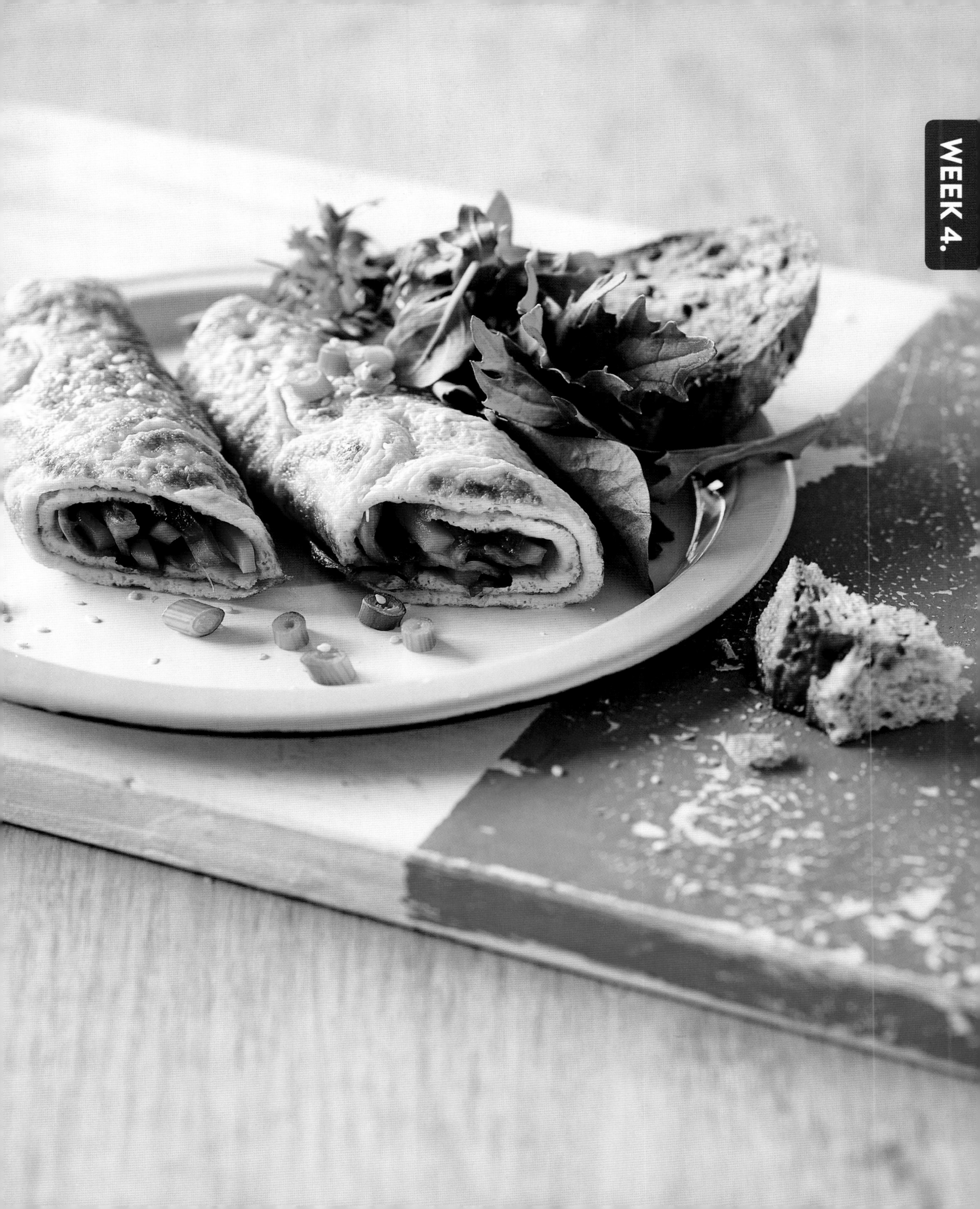

CRUNCHY GRILLED BANANA WRAP

SERVES: 2   **PREPARATION TIME:** 5 MINUTES   **COOKING TIME:** 5 MINUTES

2 small bananas

2 tablespoons peanut butter

2 tablespoons reduced-fat Greek-style yoghurt

2 wholemeal mountain bread wraps

2 tablespoons desiccated coconut, plus extra to serve

Preheat an overhead grill to high and line a baking tray with baking paper.

Slice the bananas and spread a little peanut butter over each slice. Place the banana on the prepared tray and grill for 5 minutes or until just starting to caramelise.

Spread the yoghurt over the wraps and top with the caramelised banana. Sprinkle with desiccated coconut, then roll up to enclose the filling (or leave open) and serve with a little extra coconut on the side

NUTRI DETAILS PER SERVE

345 cals/1450 kjs
Protein: 12.4 g
Fibre: 6.6 g
Total fat: 17.5 g
Sat fat: 5.9 g
Carbs: 32.3 g
Total sugar: 17.9 g
Free sugar: 0.0 g

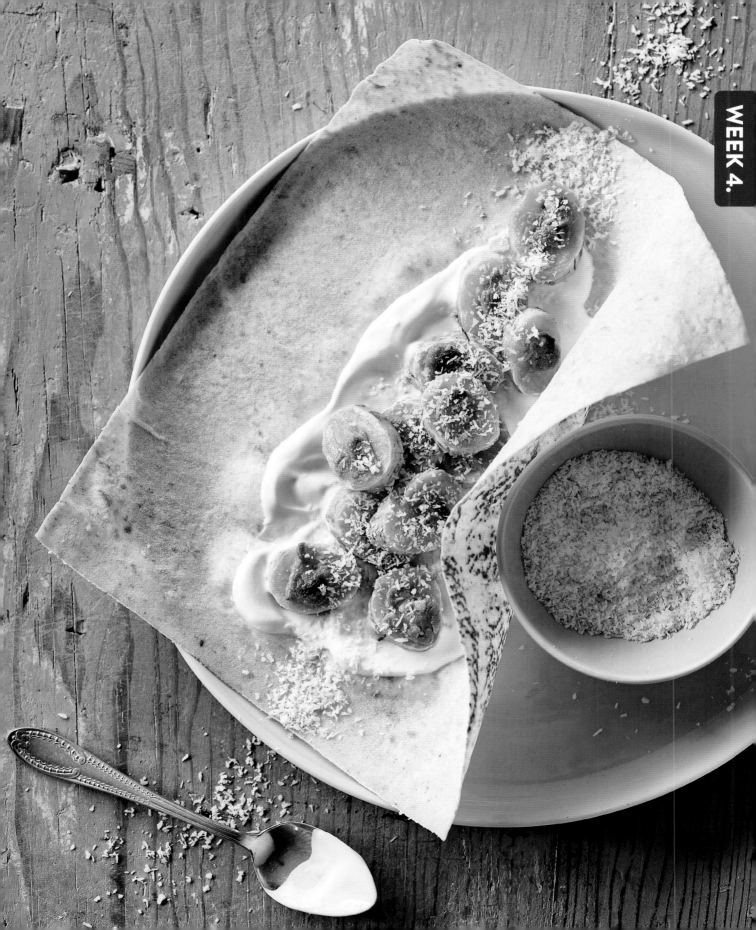

VEGGIE SCRAMBLED EGGS ON TOAST

SERVES: 2   **PREPARATION TIME:** 10 MINUTES   **COOKING TIME:** 5 MINUTES

---

2 slices wholegrain or gluten-free bread of choice

4 free-range eggs, lightly beaten

1 tomato, chopped

3 tablespoons chopped flat-leaf parsley

cooking oil spray

30 g baby spinach leaves

¾ medium avocado

NUTRI DETAILS PER SERVE

345 cals/1449 kjs
Protein: 18.8 g
Fibre: 5 g
Total fat: 22 g
Sat fat: 5.6 g
Carbs: 17 g
Total sugar: 2.7 g
Free sugar: 0.0 g

Toast the bread.

Meanwhile, whisk together the egg, tomato and parsley. Spray a medium frying pan with cooking oil spray and place over medium–high heat. Add the egg mixture and gently scrape across the pan with a flat spatula until the egg is cooked and scrambled.

Place the spinach on the toast. Slice the avocado and lay across the top of the spinach. Spoon on the scrambled egg and serve immediately.

If preferred, you could cook the spinach with the scrambled egg, or add some smoked salmon or ham for added protein.

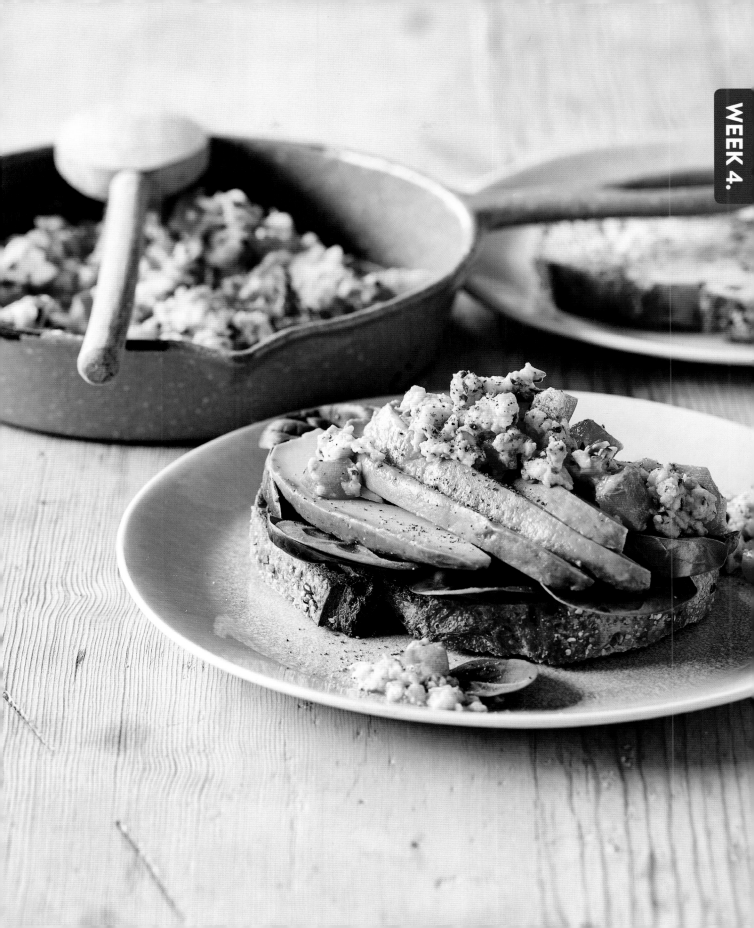

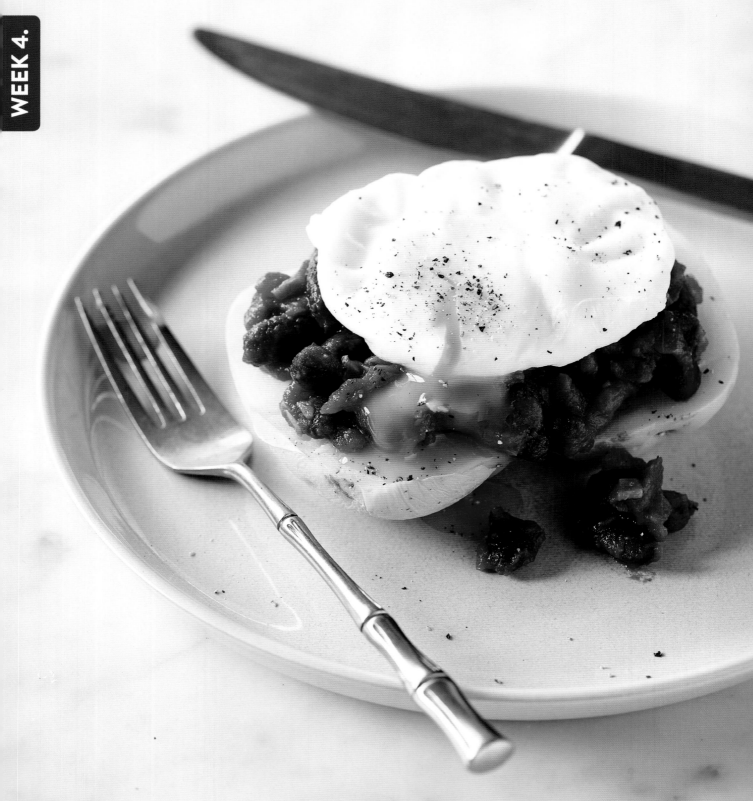

MEXICAN BREAKFAST POTATO

SERVES: 2   **PREPARATION TIME:** 10 MINUTES   **COOKING TIME:** 15 MINUTES

2 medium potatoes
2 teaspoons extra virgin olive oil
¼ red onion, diced
120 g tinned red kidney beans, drained and rinsed
⅓ cup tomato passata
1 teaspoon salt-reduced taco seasoning
2 teaspoons tomato paste
1 teaspoon white vinegar
2 free-range eggs
freshly ground black pepper

NUTRI DETAILS PER SERVE

260 cals/1088 kjs
Protein: 13.5 g
Fibre: 6.5 g
Total fat: 9.4 g
Sat fat: 1.9 g
Carbs: 25.9 g
Total sugar: 5.5 g
Free sugar: 0.0 g

Prick the potatoes all over with a fork and steam for 10 minutes or until tender.

Meanwhile, heat the olive oil in a frying pan over medium–high heat, add the onion and cook for 1–2 minutes or until translucent. Add the beans, passata, taco seasoning, tomato paste and 2 tablespoons water and simmer for 5–10 minutes or until the sauce has thickened slightly.

While the sauce is cooking, fill a medium saucepan with water until three-quarters full and bring to the boil over medium–high heat. Add the vinegar and reduce the heat to medium–low. Crack each egg into a small bowl. Use a spoon to stir the water to make a whirlpool, then carefully add one egg at a time to the centre of the whirlpool. Poach for 3 minutes for soft yolks or around 4 minutes for firm yolks. Remove the eggs with a slotted spoon.

Cut the potatoes in half and place two halves on each plate. Top with the bean sauce and poached eggs and serve sprinkled with pepper.

BANANA AND CHOC-NUT FRENCH TOAST

SERVES: 2   **PREPARATION TIME:** 10 MINUTES   **COOKING TIME:** 8 MINUTES

---

2 free-range eggs

½ teaspoon ground cinnamon

3 tablespoons reduced-fat milk of choice

4 slices wholegrain or gluten-free bread of choice

cooking oil spray

2 squares (10 g) dark chocolate (70% cocoa solids)

2 teaspoons peanut butter

1 small banana, sliced

Whisk together the eggs, cinnamon and half the milk in a shallow bowl. Dip the bread in the egg mixture and turn to coat.

Spray a non-stick frying pan with cooking oil spray and place over medium–high heat. Add the bread slices and cook for 2–3 minutes each side or until golden.

Meanwhile, gently melt the chocolate in the microwave and combine with the peanut butter. Slowly mix in the remaining milk to create a smooth sauce.

Place two slices of French toast on each plate, top with the banana slices and drizzle over the choc-nut sauce.

NUTRI DETAILS PER SERVE

369 cals/1552 kjs
Protein: 17.9 g
Fibre: 6.8 g
Total fat: 12.6 g
Sat fat: 4 g
Carbs: 43.5 g
Total sugar: 13.5 g
Free sugar: 2.7 g

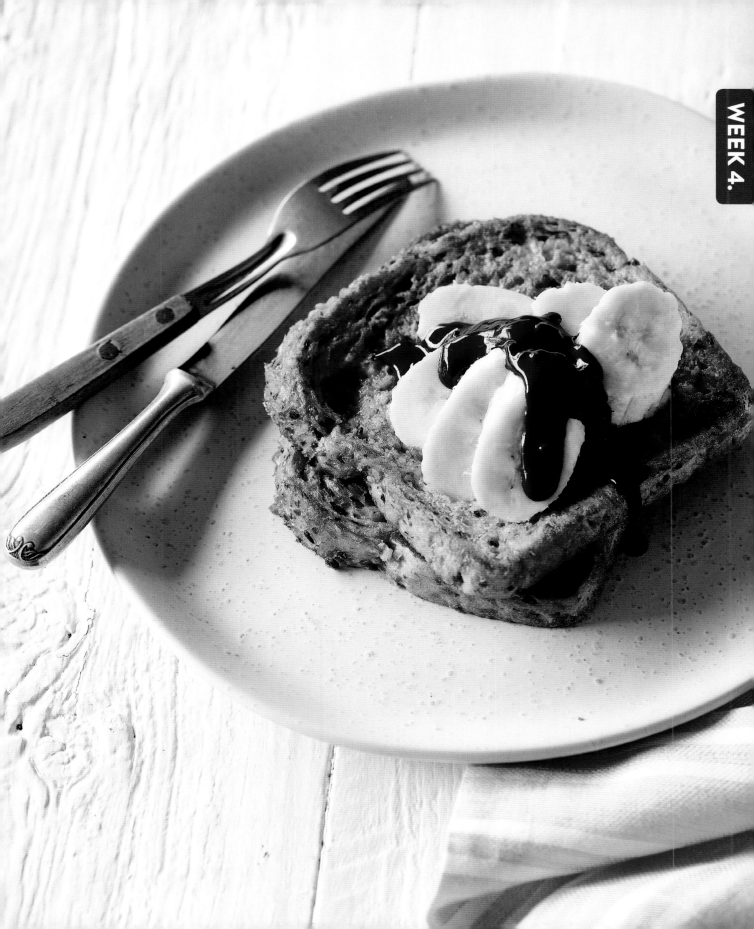

CARROT AND BEETROOT SLAW WITH HALOUMI

SERVES: 2 **PREPARATION TIME:** 10 MINUTES **COOKING TIME:** 5 MINUTES

cooking oil spray

100 g haloumi, cut into 4 slices

2 medium beetroot, peeled and grated

2 medium carrots, peeled and grated

⅓ cup chopped flat-leaf parsley leaves

2 tablespoons lemon juice

2 teaspoons extra virgin olive oil

salt and freshly ground black pepper

Lightly spray a chargrill or frying pan with cooking oil spray and place over medium–high heat. Add the haloumi slices and cook for 1–2 minutes each side or until golden.

Meanwhile, place the beetroot, carrot, parsley, lemon juice and olive oil in a bowl, season with salt and pepper, and toss to combine.

Divide the slaw between two plates, top with the haloumi slices and serve.

NUTRI DETAILS PER SERVE

336 cals/1411 kjs
Protein: 16.3 g
Fibre: 4.3 g
Total fat: 23.4 g
Sat fat: 12 g
Carbs: 17.5 g
Total sugar: 11 g
Free sugar: 0.0 g

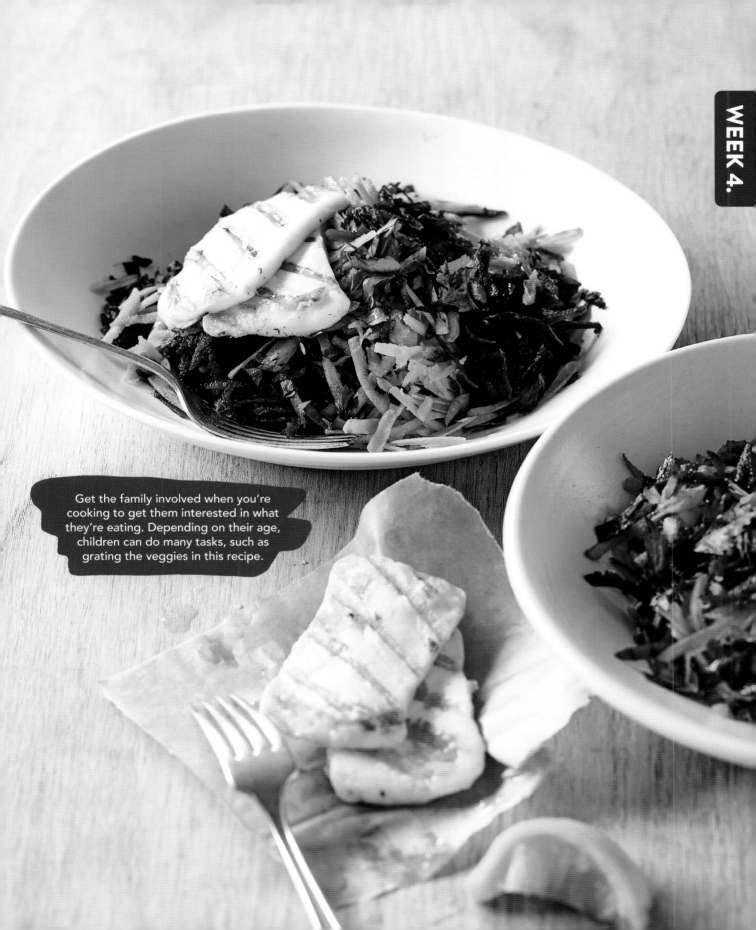

Get the family involved when you're cooking to get them interested in what they're eating. Depending on their age, children can do many tasks, such as grating the veggies in this recipe.

THICK AND CREAMY LENTIL AND TOMATO SOUP

SERVES: 2   **PREPARATION TIME:** 10 MINUTES   **COOKING TIME:** 35 MINUTES

2 teaspoons extra virgin olive oil

½ fennel bulb, trimmed and diced, fronds reserved

½ brown onion, diced

200 g tinned brown lentils, drained and rinsed

⅓ cup unsalted cashews

2 cups salt-reduced vegetable stock

½ cup tomato passata

2 teaspoons chopped flat-leaf parsley leaves

¼ teaspoon dried chilli flakes

Heat the olive oil in a medium saucepan over medium–high heat, add the fennel and onion and cook for 3–4 minutes or until softened.

Add the lentils, cashews, stock and tomato passata. Bring to the boil, then reduce the heat and simmer for 20–30 minutes. Use a stick blender or benchtop blender to blitz the soup until smooth, leaving some chunks for texture if you like.

Divide the soup between two bowls, garnish with the reserved fennel fronds, parsley and chilli and serve.

NUTRI DETAILS PER SERVE

312 cals/1312 kjs
Protein: 16.7 g
Fibre: 9.6 g
Total fat: 14 g
Sat fat: 2 g
Carbs: 26 g
Total sugar: 6.8 g
Free sugar: 0.0 g

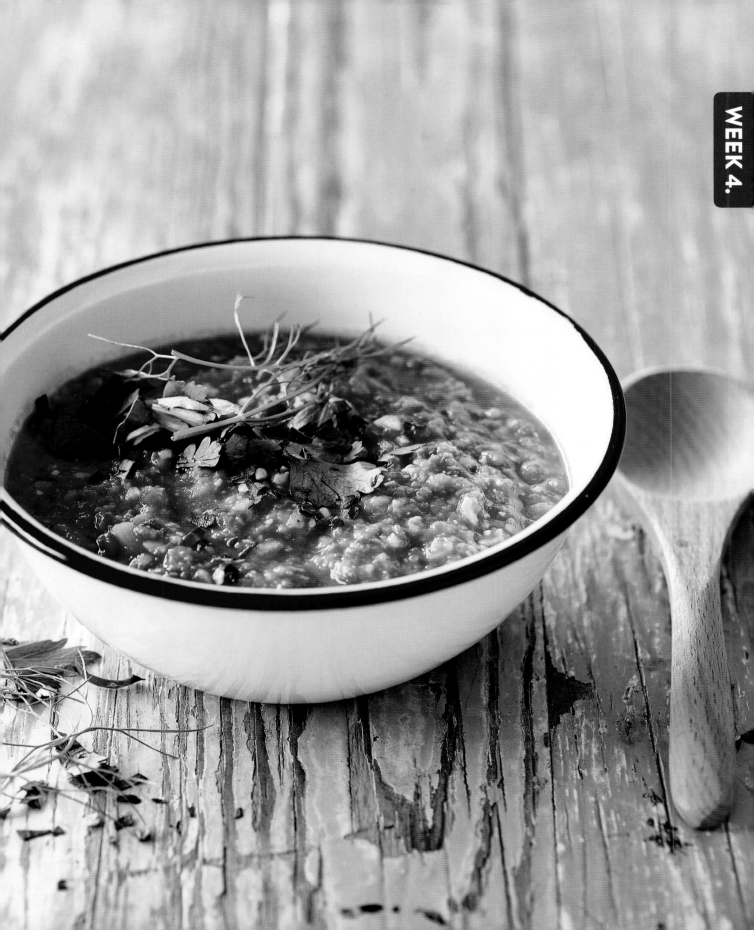

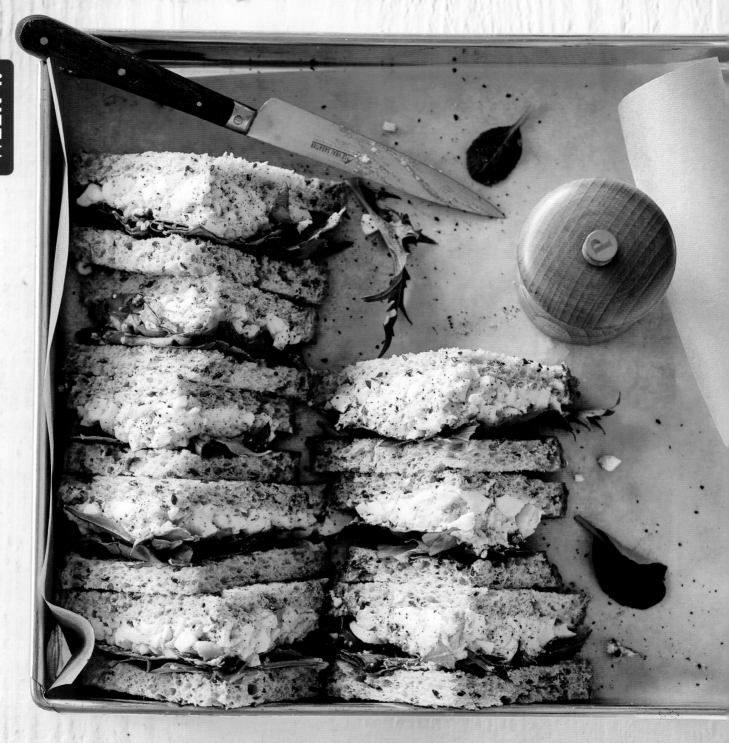

Hard-boil a few free-range eggs at the beginning of every week and store them in an airtight container in the fridge. They can be used in recipes like this one, and also make an easy-to-grab, healthy snack.

HEALTHY EGG SANDWICHES

SERVES: 2   **PREPARATION TIME:** 5 MINUTES   **COOKING TIME:** 10 MINUTES

4 hard-boiled free-range eggs, peeled

1 tablespoon reduced-fat mayonnaise

salt and freshly ground black pepper

4 slices wholegrain or gluten-free bread of choice

30 g mixed lettuce leaves

Mash together the hard-boiled eggs and mayonnaise, and season with salt and pepper.

Place two slices of bread on a board and spread evenly with the egg mixture. Top with the lettuce leaves, then sandwich with the remaining bread slices and serve, cut diagonally into quarters if desired.

NUTRI DETAILS PER SERVE

345 cals/1453 kjs
Protein: 20.3 g
Fibre: 5.3 g
Total fat: 13.8 g
Sat fat: 3.6 g
Carbs: 32 g
Total sugar: 3.6 g
Free sugar: 0.0 g

LIME AND COCONUT CHICKEN RICE

SERVES: 2   **PREPARATION TIME:** 10 MINUTES   **COOKING TIME:** 45 MINUTES

½ cup brown rice

cooking oil spray

160 g chicken breast fillets

2 tablespoons coconut cream

2 tablespoons lime juice

1 tablespoon fish sauce

60 g cos lettuce leaves, roughly chopped

3 tablespoons mint leaves

salt and freshly ground black pepper

NUTRI DETAILS PER SERVE

350 cals/1472 kjs
Protein: 22.7 g
Fibre: 2.8 g
Total fat: 9.9 g
Sat fat: 5.2 g
Carbs: 40.6 g
Total sugar: 2.2 g
Free sugar: 0.0 g

Bring 2 cups water to the boil in a medium saucepan, add the rice and simmer for 45 minutes or until tender. Drain. You could use pre-cooked rice for this recipe if you have some on hand. Just warm it through first.

Meanwhile, spray a non-stick frying pan with cooking oil spray and place over medium heat. Add the chicken breast fillets and cook for 4–5 minutes each side or until nicely browned and cooked through. Leave to cool, then slice or shred the meat. As with the rice, you could use pre-cooked shredded chicken if you have some.

Mix together the coconut cream, lime juice and fish sauce to make the dressing.

Place the chicken, lettuce and mint in a bowl and toss with half the dressing.

Divide the rice and chicken salad between two plates and drizzle over the remaining dressing. Season with salt and pepper and serve.

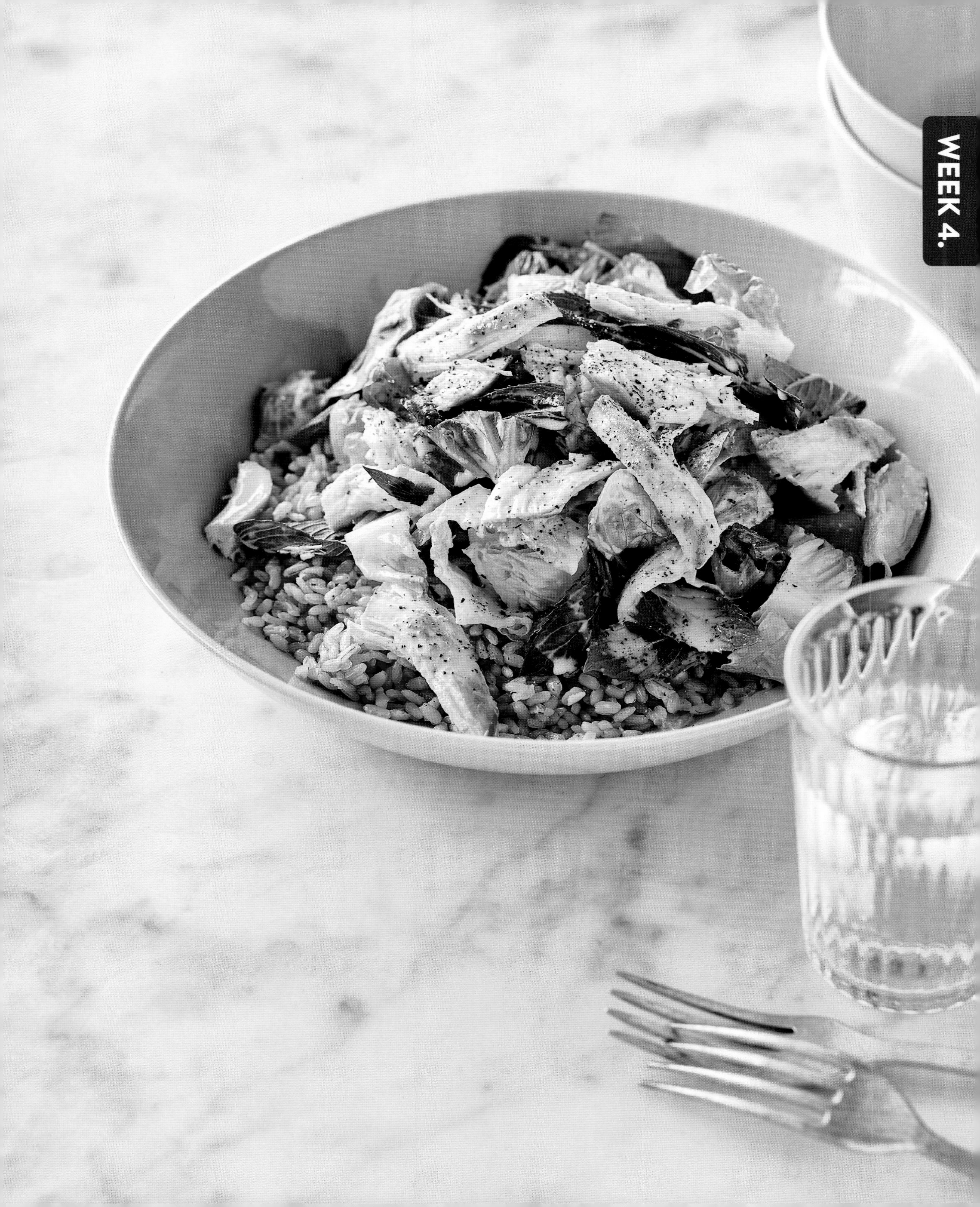

CHILLI, TUNA AND AVOCADO OPEN SANDWICH

SERVES: 2   **PREPARATION TIME:** 10 MINUTES   **COOKING TIME:** 5 MINUTES

180 g tinned tuna in spring water, drained

⅔ medium avocado

1 spring onion, finely sliced

2 tablespoons reduced-fat Greek-style yoghurt

1 tablespoon lemon juice

½ teaspoon dried chilli flakes

2 slices wholegrain or gluten-free bread of choice

30 g rocket leaves

Place the tuna, avocado, spring onion, yoghurt, lemon juice and chilli flakes in a bowl and mash well to combine.

Toast the bread and spread evenly with the tuna and avocado mixture. Top with the rocket leaves and serve.

NUTRI DETAILS PER SERVE

306 cals/1285 kjs
Protein: 27.9 g
Fibre: 4.6 g
Total fat: 9.9 g
Sat fat: 2.1 g
Carbs: 29.4 g
Total sugar: 5.6 g
Free sugar: 0.0 g

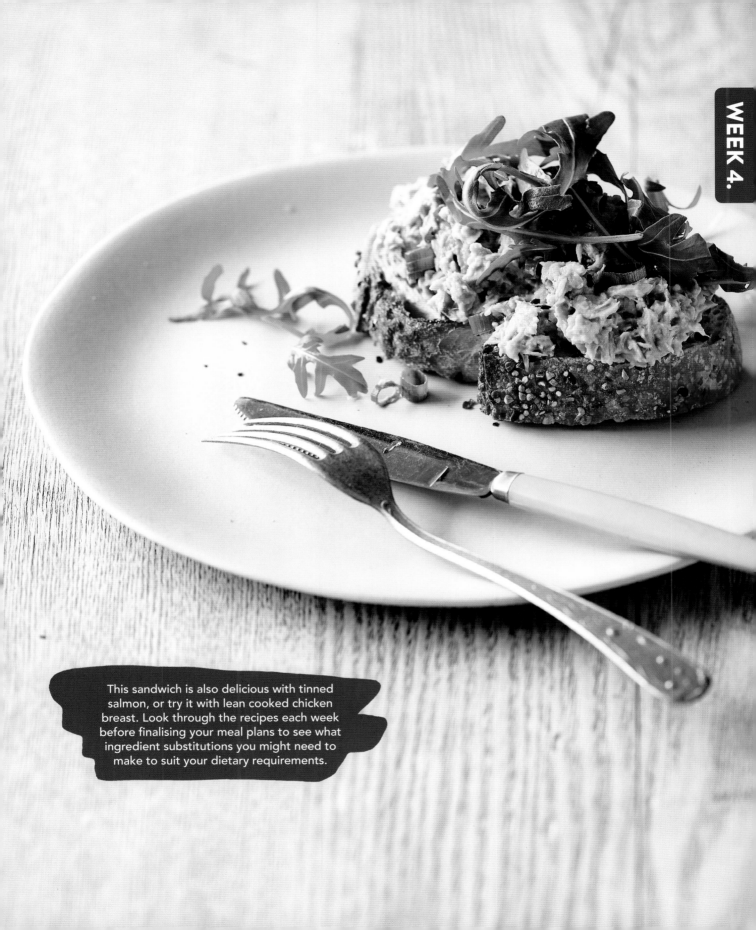

This sandwich is also delicious with tinned salmon, or try it with lean cooked chicken breast. Look through the recipes each week before finalising your meal plans to see what ingredient substitutions you might need to make to suit your dietary requirements.

OCHAZUKE

SERVES: 2   **PREPARATION TIME:** 10 MINUTES   **COOKING TIME:** 20 MINUTES

1 cup sushi rice

2 green teabags

1 cup boiling water

1 medium carrot, finely sliced

1 nori sheet, finely sliced

40 g mushrooms, sliced

2 tablespoons chopped flat-leaf parsley leaves

1 tablespoon black or white sesame seeds

2 teaspoons salt-reduced soy sauce

Rinse the rice in a colander until the water runs clear. Place in a medium saucepan with 1½ cups water and bring to the boil. Reduce the heat to low and cook, covered, for 20 minutes or until the rice is tender and has absorbed the water.

Meanwhile, place the teabags in a cup and pour over the boiling water. Allow to steep for a couple of minutes.

Divide the rice between two bowls and top with the carrot, nori, mushroom, parsley and sesame seeds. Pour the green tea over the top to create a broth, then drizzle with the soy sauce and serve.

NUTRI DETAILS PER SERVE

362 cals/1516 kjs
Protein: 9.4 g
Fibre: 5.4 g
Total fat: 5.1 g
Sat fat: 0.6 g
Carbs: 66 g
Total sugar: 2.1 g
Free sugar: 0.0 g

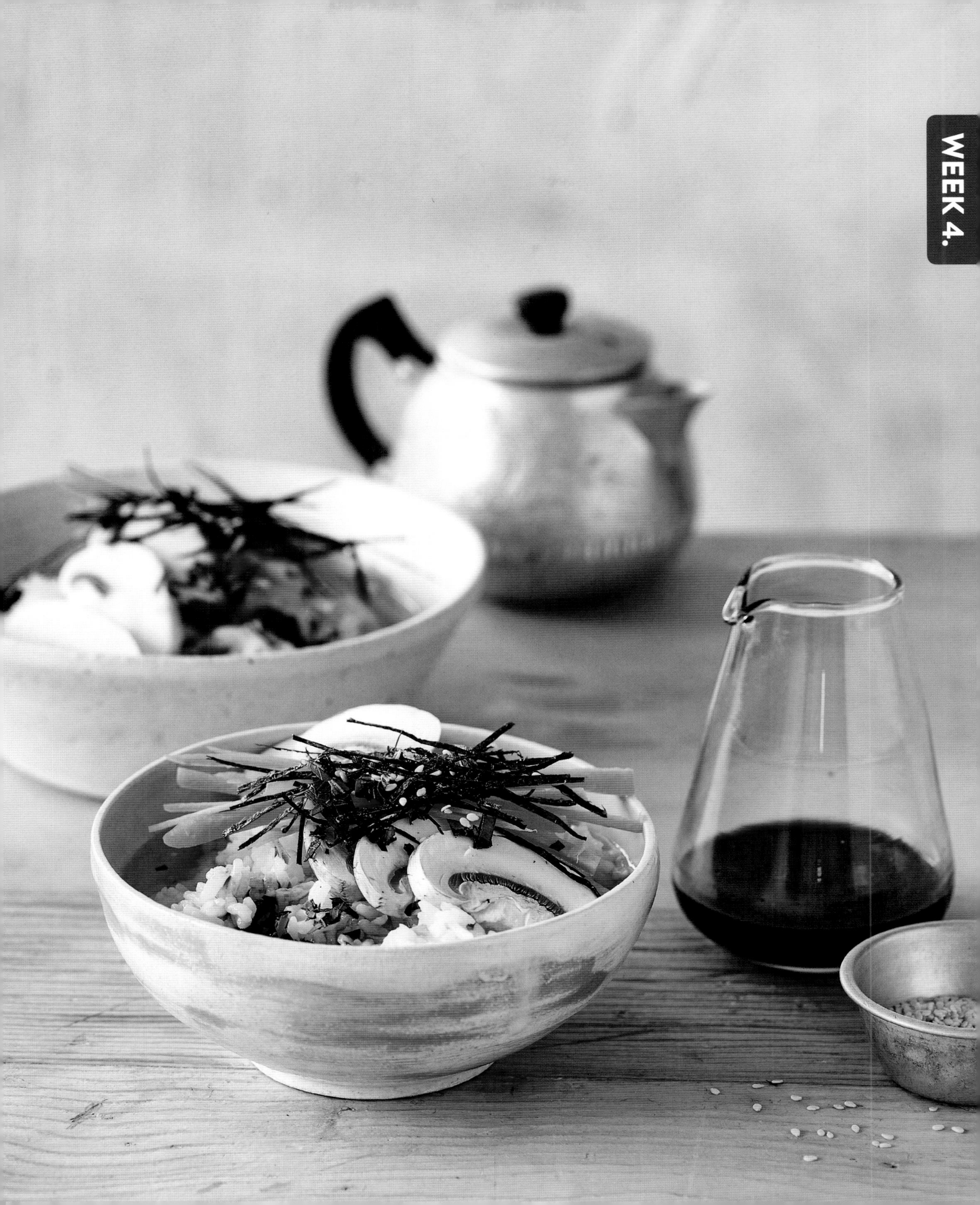

When freezing leftovers or extra meals remember to label and date them so you know what is inside your containers. You don't want all your fantastic meal prep going to waste!

PUMPKIN, BACON AND SWEET POTATO SOUP

SERVES: 2   **PREPARATION TIME:** 10 MINUTES   **COOKING TIME:** 25 MINUTES

20 g butter

1 brown onion, chopped

2 garlic cloves, finely chopped

450 g pumpkin, peeled, seeds removed and cut into 2 cm cubes

1 small sweet potato, peeled and cut into 2 cm cubes

1 cup salt-reduced chicken stock

½ teaspoon dried basil

200 ml reduced-fat coconut milk

2 lean bacon rashers, trimmed

freshly ground black pepper

Melt the butter in a medium saucepan over medium–high heat, add the onion, garlic, pumpkin and sweet potato and cook for 5 minutes or until the onion has softened. Add the stock and basil and simmer for 10–15 minutes or until the vegetables are very tender. Pour in the coconut milk and cook for a further 5 minutes.

While the soup is simmering, cook the bacon in a non-stick frying pan for 5 minutes or until crispy. Chop into pieces and set aside.

Use a stick blender or benchtop blender to blitz the soup until smooth. Return to the heat to gently warm through if required.

Divide the soup between two bowls and top with the bacon pieces. Season with freshly ground black pepper and serve.

NUTRI DETAILS PER SERVE

269 cals/1133 kjs

Protein: 10.6 g

Fibre: 3.6 g

Total fat: 13.5 g

Sat fat: 4.9 g

Carbs: 25.3 g

Total sugar: 12 g

Free sugar: 0.0 g

PORK WITH TANGY COLESLAW

SERVES: 4   **PREPARATION TIME:** 10 MINUTES   **COOKING TIME:** 15 MINUTES

cooking oil spray
600 g pork fillet
salt and freshly ground black
   pepper
200 g white cabbage, shredded
4 medium carrots, grated
⅔ cup chopped flat-leaf parsley
   leaves
½ cup reduced-fat mayonnaise
⅓ cup lemon juice

Lightly spray a medium frying pan with cooking oil spray and place over medium–high heat. Season the pork with salt and pepper on all sides, then add to the pan and cook for 5–7 minutes each side or until cooked through. Transfer the pork to a plate and allow to rest while you make the coleslaw.

Combine the cabbage, carrot, parsley, mayonnaise and lemon juice in a bowl.

Slice the pork and divide among four plates. Serve with the coleslaw on the side.

NUTRI DETAILS PER SERVE

295 cals/1237 kjs
Protein: 35.6 g
Fibre: 4.3 g
Total fat: 10.6 g
Sat fat: 2 g
Carbs: 13.7 g
Total sugar: 11 g
Free sugar: 0.0 g

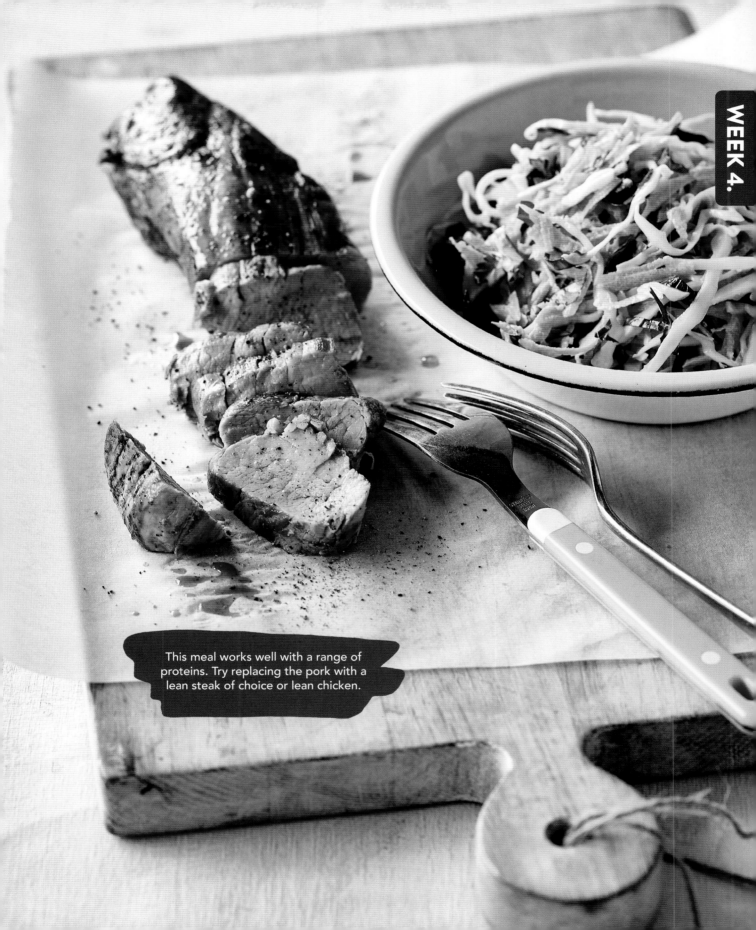

This meal works well with a range of proteins. Try replacing the pork with a lean steak of choice or lean chicken.

SPANISH RICE WITH CHORIZO

SERVES: 4   **PREPARATION TIME:** 10 MINUTES   **COOKING TIME:** 45 MINUTES

1 cup brown rice

2 chorizo sausages, chopped

1 brown onion, diced

4 tomatoes, diced

1 cup frozen peas

1 cup corn kernels (fresh or tinned)

1 red capsicum, seeds removed, diced

1 teaspoon smoked paprika

1 tablespoon chopped flat-leaf parsley leaves

4 lime wedges

Bring 1 litre water to the boil in a medium saucepan, add the rice and simmer for 45 minutes or until tender. Drain.

Meanwhile, heat a non-stick frying pan over medium heat, add the chorizo and cook on both sides for 3 minutes or until the edges are crisp. Transfer to a plate lined with paper towel and set aside.

Add the onion to the pan and cook for 2 minutes or until it starts to turn golden. Add the tomato, peas, corn, capsicum and paprika and toss to combine. Cook for 3 minutes or until the vegetables are just tender.

Add the cooked rice and return the chorizo to the pan, then toss together well. Divide among four plates, garnish with the parsley and serve with lime wedges.

NUTRI DETAILS PER SERVE

409 cals/1710 kjs
Protein: 20 g
Fibre: 8.4 g
Total fat: 13.7 g
Sat fat: 4.3 g
Carbs: 46 g
Total sugar: 7.2 g
Free sugar: 0.0 g

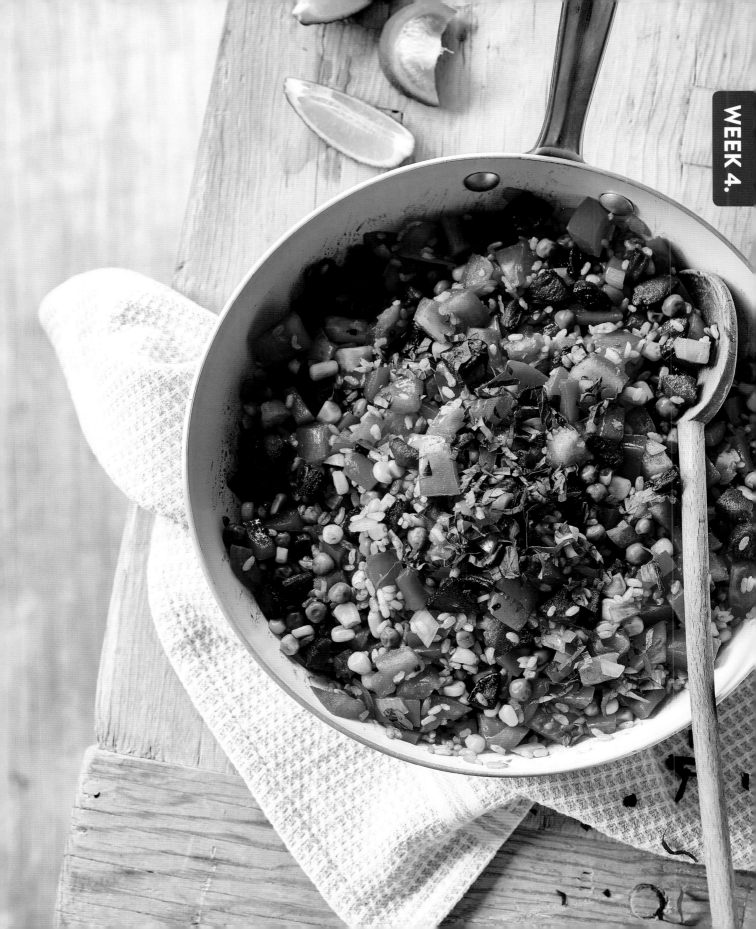

SPICY BEEF AND BLACK BEAN SALAD

SERVES: 4   **PREPARATION TIME:** 10 MINUTES   **COOKING TIME:** 10 MINUTES

2 teaspoons ground cumin

2 teaspoons chilli powder

320 g lean sirloin steak

cooking oil spray

240 g tinned black beans, drained and rinsed

2 cup corn kernels (fresh or tinned)

1 red capsicum, seeds removed, diced

4 spring onions, finely sliced

4 tomatoes, diced

2 teaspoons extra virgin olive oil

1 tablespoon lemon juice

Sprinkle the cumin and chilli powder over the steak.

Lightly spray a frying pan with cooking oil spray and place over medium–high heat. Add the steak and cook for 2–3 minutes each side or until cooked to your liking. Set aside to rest while you make the salad.

Combine the black beans, corn, capsicum, spring onion and tomato in a bowl. Dress with the olive oil and lemon juice and gently toss to coat.

Divide the salad among four plates. Thinly slice the steak and place on top of the salad to serve.

NUTRI DETAILS PER SERVE

308 cals/1291 kjs
Protein: 29 g
Fibre: 11.8 g
Total fat: 8.2 g
Sat fat: 2.1 g
Carbs: 23 g
Total sugar: 7.2 g
Free sugar: 0.0 g

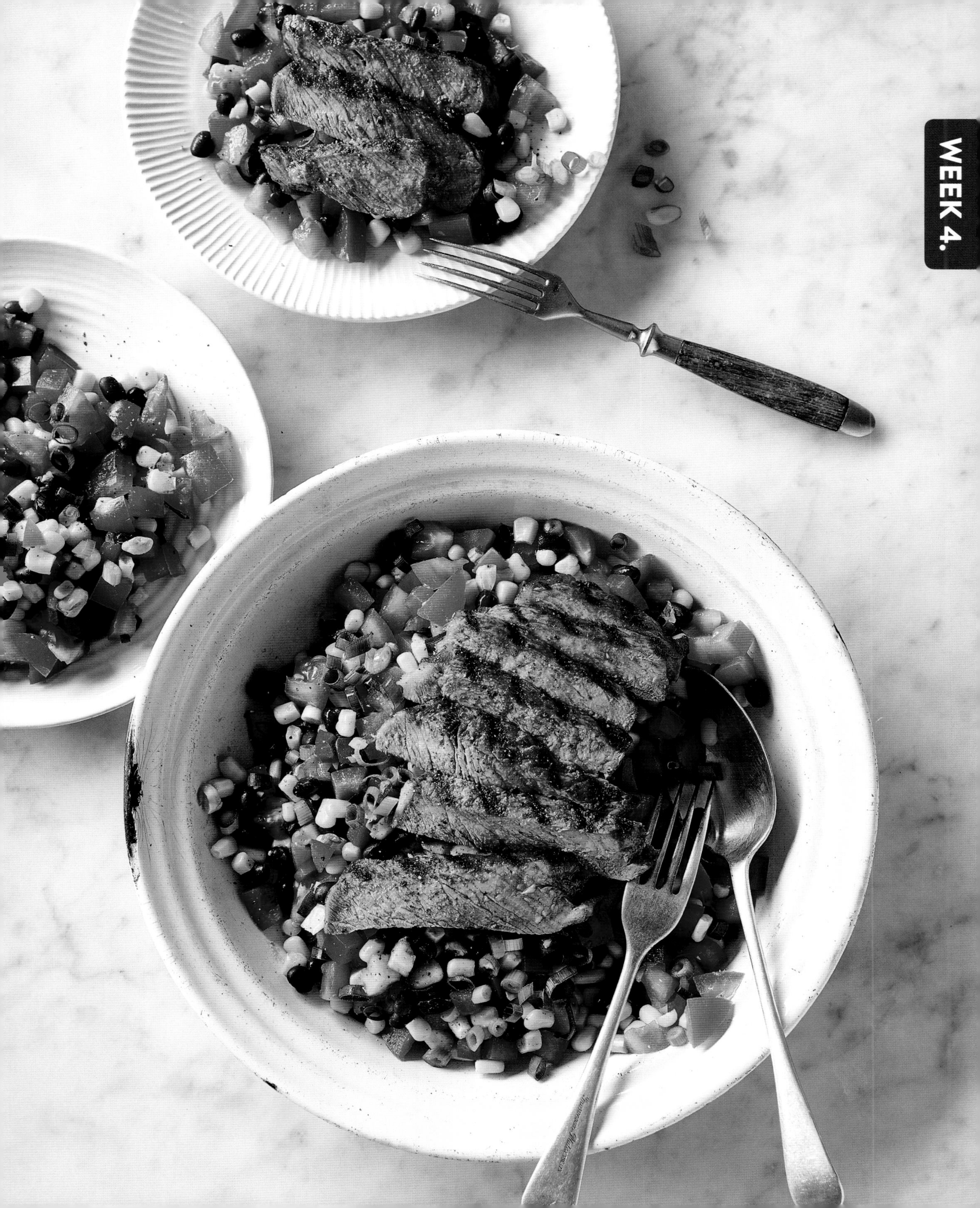

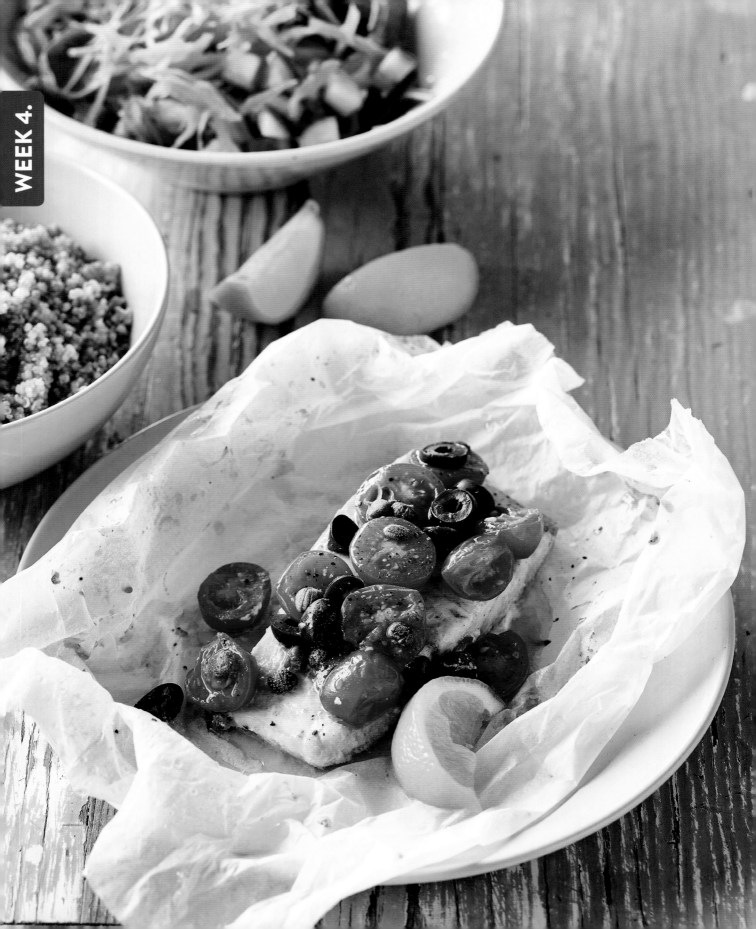

FISH WITH OLIVE AND CHILLI SAUCE

SERVES: 4   **PREPARATION TIME:** 15 MINUTES   **COOKING TIME:** 20 MINUTES

4 × 150 g white fish fillets of choice, skin and bones removed
350 g cherry tomatoes, halved
⅔ cup kalamata olives, pitted
2 bird's eye chillies, sliced
1 tablespoon baby capers
1 tablespoon extra virgin olive oil
salt and freshly ground black pepper
1 cup quinoa
120 g baby spinach leaves
2 medium carrots, grated
1 Lebanese cucumber, diced
2 tablespoons lemon juice
lemon wedges, to serve

Preheat the oven to 180°C.

Place each portion of fish on a square of baking paper on a large baking tray and top evenly with the tomatoes, olives, chilli and capers. Drizzle with half the olive oil and season with salt and pepper. Wrap the baking paper around the fish and vegetables to form four parcels and bake for 15–20 minutes or until the fish is cooked through and the tomatoes have collapsed.

Meanwhile, place the quinoa and 2 cups water in a saucepan and bring to the boil. Reduce the heat and simmer, covered, for 15 minutes or until tender and most of the liquid has been absorbed. Fluff up with a fork.

Combine the baby spinach, carrot and cucumber in a bowl. Dress with the lemon juice and remaining olive oil and gently toss to coat.

Divide the quinoa among four plates and top with the fish, tomatoes, olives and capers. Drizzle over any cooking juices from the parcels and serve with the salad and lemon wedges.

NUTRI DETAILS PER SERVE

228 cals/957 kjs
Protein: 11.7 g
Fibre: 4.8 g
Total fat: 12.3 g
Sat fat: 1.6 g
Carbs: 15.8 g
Total sugar: 4.9 g
Free sugar: 0.0 g

ULTIMATE BEAN NACHOS

SERVES: 4   **PREPARATION TIME:** 15 MINUTES   **COOKING TIME:** 5 MINUTES

4 wholemeal mountain bread wraps

cooking oil spray

140 g tinned red kidney beans, drained and rinsed

1 tablespoon tomato paste

salt and freshly ground black pepper

1 medium avocado

4 spring onions, chopped

1 red capsicum, seeds removed, finely chopped

2 tomatoes, chopped

2 teaspoons lemon juice

⅓ cup coriander leaves

⅓ cup grated reduced-fat cheddar

⅓ cup reduced-fat Greek-style yoghurt

Preheat an overhead grill to high. Cut the mountain bread wraps in half, then quarters, and then into triangles. Spray with cooking oil spray, place on a baking tray and grill for 30 seconds each side or until crisp and golden.

Mash the kidney beans and place in a saucepan with the tomato paste and 1 tablespoon water. Stir over medium heat to warm through, then remove from the heat and cover and keep warm (add a little extra water if the mixture is too thick). Season to taste with salt and pepper.

Mash the avocado in a bowl, then stir in the spring onion, capsicum, tomato and lemon juice. Season with salt and pepper.

Divide the mountain bread chips among four plates. Top with the beans, avocado mixture, coriander, cheese and yoghurt, and serve.

NUTRI DETAILS PER SERVE

415 cals/1743 kjs
Protein: 19.5 g
Fibre: 10.4 g
Total fat: 17.2 g
Sat fat: 7.2 g
Carbs: 47.5 g
Total sugar: 6 g
Free sugar: 0.0 g

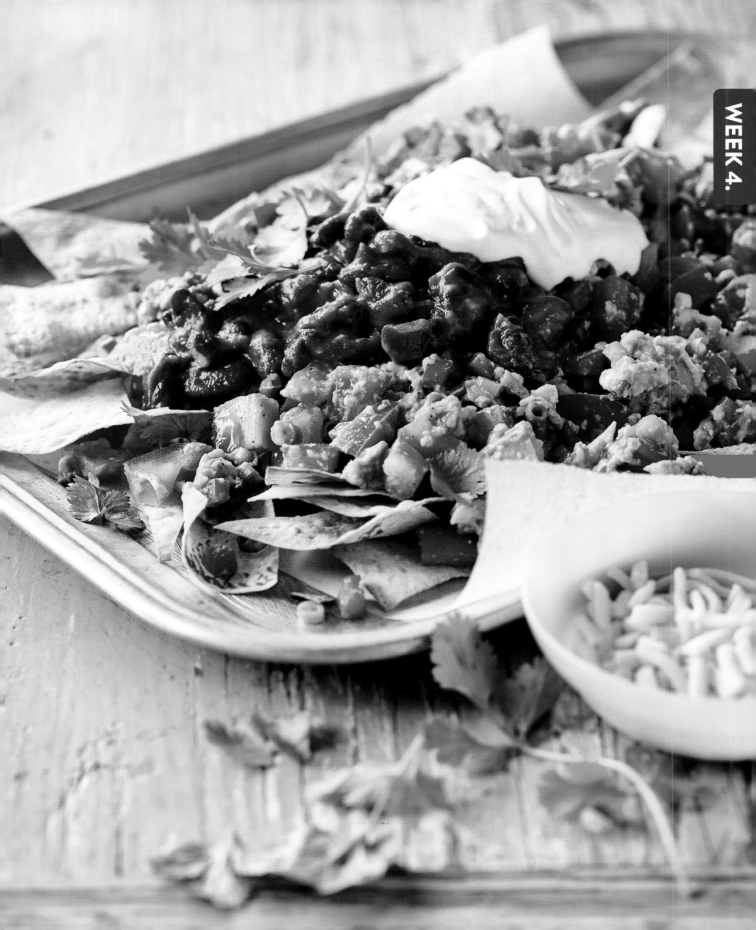

THAI CALAMARI SALAD

SERVES: 4 **PREPARATION TIME:** 15 MINUTES, PLUS MARINATING AND SOAKING TIME
COOKING TIME: 15 MINUTES

---

600 g calamari (fresh or frozen and thawed), cleaned and cut into rings

½ cup chopped coriander leaves

⅓ cup sweet chilli sauce

2 tablespoons lime juice

130 g rice vermicelli noodles

2 medium carrots, finely sliced or grated

1 Lebanese cucumber, finely sliced

120 g mixed lettuce leaves

2 tablespoons sesame oil

2 bird's eye chillies, sliced

Combine the calamari, coriander, sweet chilli sauce and lime juice in a bowl, then set aside to marinate for at least 15 minutes.

Meanwhile, place the noodles in a heatproof bowl and cover with boiling water. Allow to soak for 10 minutes or until the noodles are tender. Drain well.

Place the noodles, carrot, cucumber and lettuce leaves in a bowl and toss gently to combine.

Heat the sesame oil in a frying pan over high heat, add the calamari and marinade and quickly pan-fry for just a minute or two each side.

Divide the noodle salad among four plates, place the calamari on top and pour over any remaining pan juices. Top with the sliced chilli and serve.

NUTRI DETAILS PER SERVE

286 cals/1200 kjs
Protein: 27 g
Fibre: 3.1 g
Total fat: 11.3 g
Sat fat: 1.9 g
Carbs: 17.4 g
Total sugar: 8.8 g
Free sugar: 0.0 g

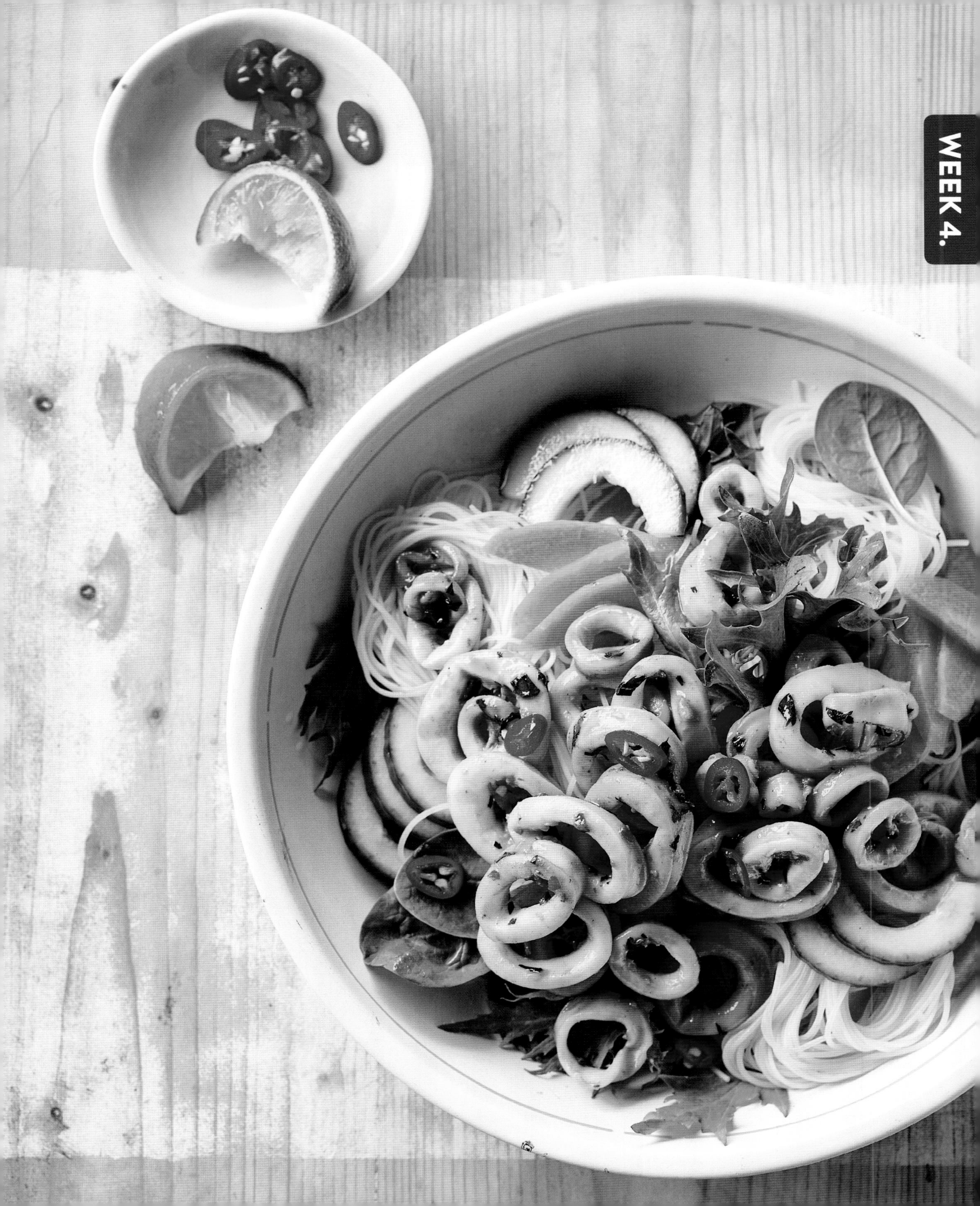

SATAY FRIED RICE WITH EGG

SERVES: 4   **PREPARATION TIME:** 10 MINUTES   **COOKING TIME:** 55 MINUTES

1 cup brown rice
⅓ cup peanut butter
2 teaspoons salt-reduced soy
  sauce
cooking oil spray
2 medium carrots, diced
1 cup frozen peas
2 spring onions, sliced
2 teaspoons sesame oil
4 free-range eggs
120 g rocket leaves

NUTRI DETAILS PER SERVE

433 cals/1818 kjs
Protein: 19 g
Fibre: 8 g
Total fat: 21 g
Sat fat: 4 g
Carbs: 40 g
Total sugar: 5 g
Free sugar: 0.0 g

Bring 1 litre water to the boil in a medium saucepan, add the rice and simmer for 45 minutes or until tender. Drain.

Place the peanut butter, soy sauce and ⅓ cup water in a bowl and stir until smooth. Set aside.

Spray a wok or frying pan with cooking oil spray and place over medium heat. Add the carrot and a splash of water and stir-fry for 5 minutes or until just tender.

Add the peas and spring onion and toss to combine, then add the rice and stir-fry for 1 minute to warm through. Add the peanut butter mixture and stir to coat the rice and veggies.

Push the rice mixture to one side of the pan and add the sesame oil to the other side. Crack the eggs into the oil and scramble lightly, then fold them through the rice mixture.

Divide the fried rice among four bowls and serve with the rocket.

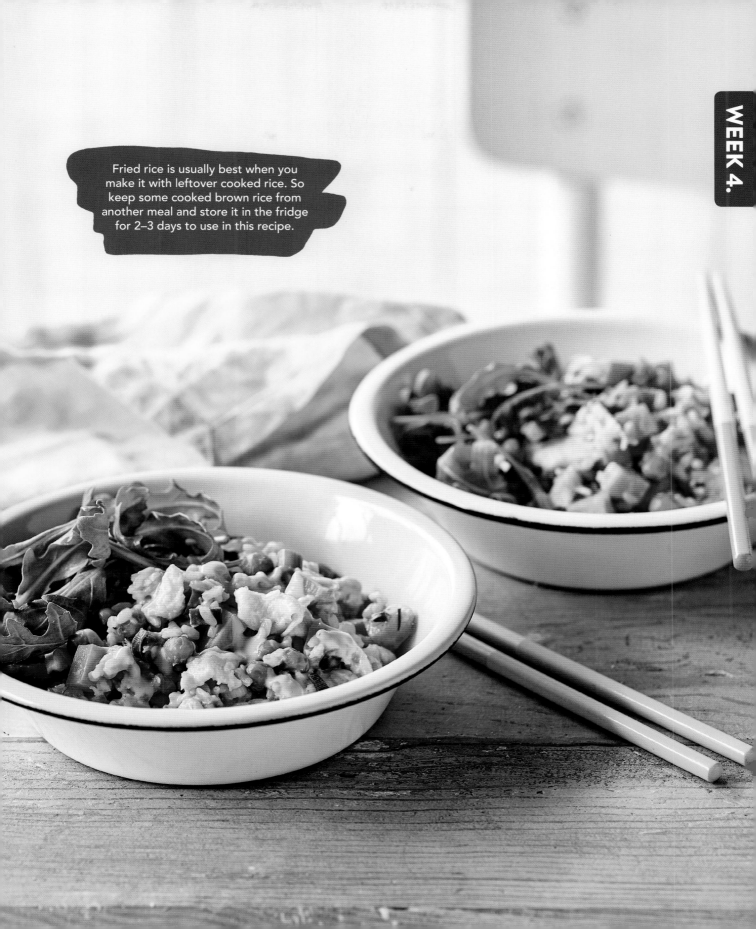

Fried rice is usually best when you make it with leftover cooked rice. So keep some cooked brown rice from another meal and store it in the fridge for 2–3 days to use in this recipe.

CHOCOLATE PEANUT BUTTER CRUMBLE BALLS

SERVES: 5 **PREPARATION TIME:** 10 MINUTES, PLUS SOAKING TIME

½ cup pitted dried dates
boiling water, for soaking
½ cup rolled oats
2 tablespoons peanut butter
2 teaspoons cacao/cocoa powder
1 ½ tablespoons desiccated coconut

Soak the dates in boiling water for 15 minutes, then drain.

Place the dates, rolled oats, peanut butter and cacao/cocoa powder in a blender and blitz until well combined. Roll the mixture into 10 even balls, then roll the balls in the desiccated coconut to coat.

Two balls is one serve. Store leftovers in an airtight container in the fridge for 3 days or freeze for up to 3 months.

NUTRI DETAILS PER SERVE

154 cals/647 kjs
Protein: 4 g
Fibre: 3.3 g
Total fat: 7.7 g
Sat fat: 2.4 g
Carbs: 16.4 g
Total sugar: 11.3 g
Free sugar: 0.0 g

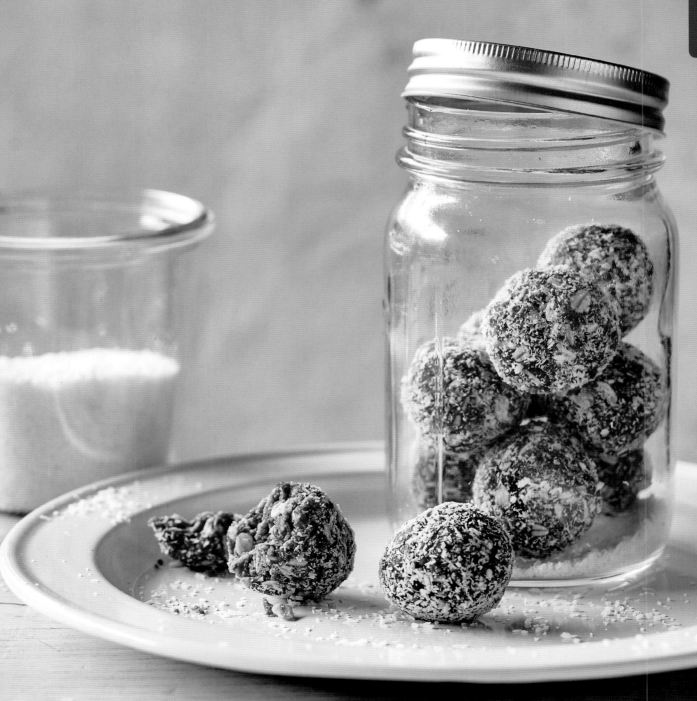

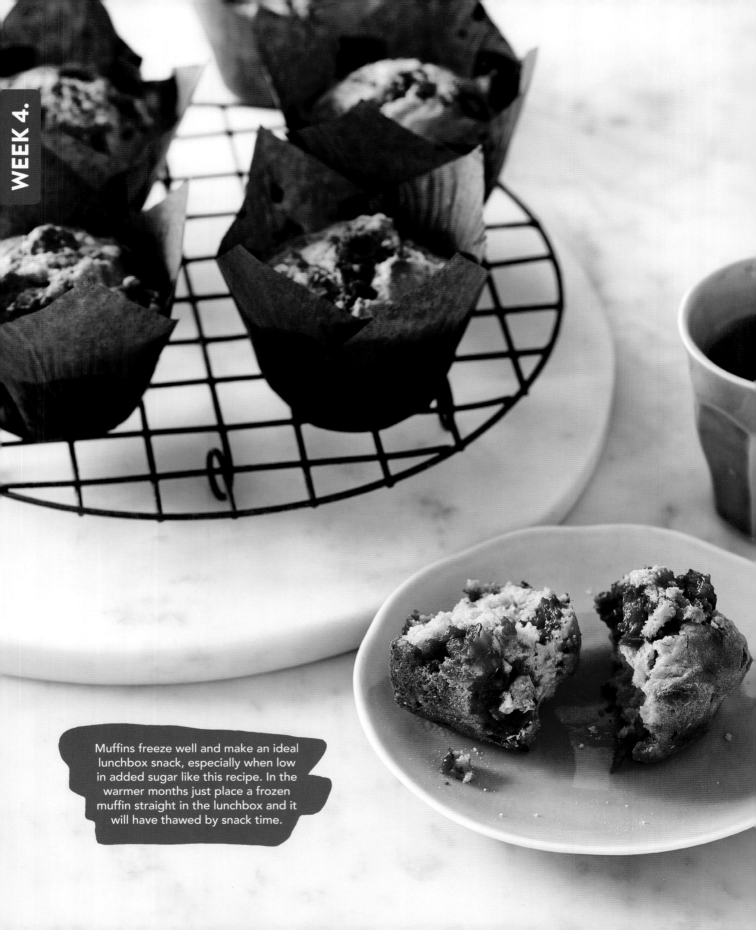

Muffins freeze well and make an ideal lunchbox snack, especially when low in added sugar like this recipe. In the warmer months just place a frozen muffin straight in the lunchbox and it will have thawed by snack time.

RASPBERRY MUFFINS

SERVES: 6   **PREPARATION TIME:** 10 MINUTES   **COOKING TIME:** 25 MINUTES

cooking oil spray

1 ⅓ cups plain wholemeal flour

½ teaspoon baking powder

1 cup fresh or frozen raspberries

2 free-range eggs

3 tablespoons reduced-fat milk of choice

60 g butter, melted

2 tablespoons honey

1 teaspoon finely grated lemon zest

Preheat the oven to 180°C. Lightly spray six standard muffin holes with cooking oil spray or line with paper patty cases.

Sift the flour and baking powder into a bowl. Stir through the raspberries to coat well.

Lightly whisk together the eggs, milk, butter, honey and lemon zest. Add to the flour mixture and stir briefly just to combine – don't overmix the batter or the muffins will be tough.

Spoon the batter evenly into the muffin holes and bake for 20–22 minutes or until a skewer inserted in the centre comes out clean.

One serve is one muffin. Store leftovers in an airtight container in the fridge for 3–4 days or freeze for up to 2 months.

NUTRI DETAILS PER SERVE

231 cals/969 kjs
Protein: 6 g
Fibre: 4 g
Total fat: 11 g
Sat fat: 6 g
Carbs: 26 g
Total sugar: 10 g
Free sugar: 5.5 g

CHEESE AND CHILLI CHIPS WITH HERBY YOGHURT DIP

SERVES: 3   **PREPARATION TIME:** 10 MINUTES, PLUS COOLING TIME   **COOKING TIME:** 10 MINUTES

½ cup grated reduced-fat cheddar

3 tablespoons grated parmesan

1 teaspoon dried chilli flakes

½ cup reduced-fat Greek-style yoghurt

1 garlic clove, minced

2 tablespoons mixed chopped herbs, such as basil, flat-leaf parsley and chives

2 teaspoons extra virgin olive oil

NUTRI DETAILS PER SERVE

144 cals/604 kjs
Protein: 11.1 g
Fibre: 0.5 g
Total fat: 9.2 g
Sat fat: 4.3 g
Carbs: 3.5 g
Total sugar: 3.4 g
Free sugar: 0.0 g

Preheat the oven to 180°C and line two baking trays with baking paper.

Combine the cheeses and chilli flakes in a bowl. Carefully spoon the mixture into 12 flat piles on the prepared trays.

Bake for 10 minutes. Watch the chips carefully as they can overcook and burn quite quickly.

Cool on the trays for 15 minutes before serving.

Place the yoghurt, garlic, herbs and olive oil in a bowl and mix well.

Divide the dip into three portions and serve each portion with four cheese chips. Any leftover dip will keep in an airtight container in the fridge for 3–4 days. Store leftover chips in an airtight container in the pantry for 3–4 days.

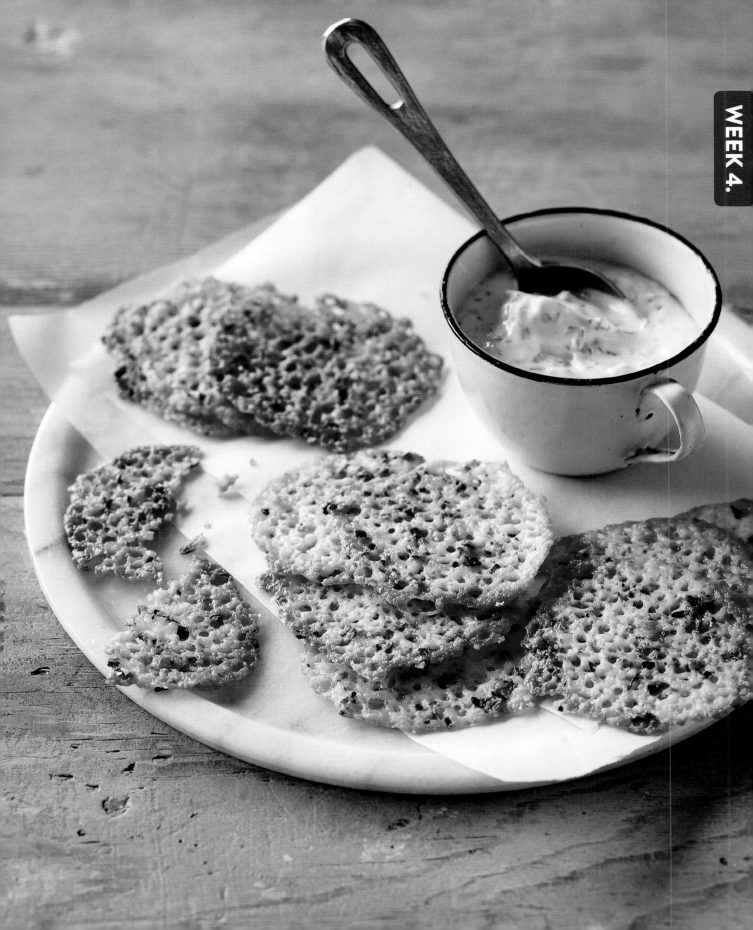

LAYERED YOGHURT AND RASPBERRY SORBET

SERVES: 8   **PREPARATION TIME:** 15 MINUTES, PLUS FREEZING TIME

1 cup reduced-fat Greek-style yoghurt

1 tablespoon honey

½ teaspoon vanilla extract

1 small banana

½ teaspoon ground cinnamon

2 tablespoons pure maple syrup

300 g fresh or frozen raspberries (thaw if frozen)

2 tablespoons mint leaves

NUTRI DETAILS PER SERVE

83 cals/351 kjs

Protein: 2.4 g

Fibre: 2.9 g

Total fat: 0.7 g

Sat fat: 0.3 g

Carbs: 14.9 g

Total sugar: 13.9 g

Free sugar: 7 g

Combine the yoghurt, honey, vanilla, banana and cinnamon in a food processor and process until smooth. Pour the mixture evenly into the base of eight silicone muffin moulds, about three quarters full. (Silicone works best but you could also line a regular muffin tin with paper cases or baking paper for easy removal.) Cover and place in the freezer for 2 hours or until frozen.

Once the yoghurt mixture is frozen, prepare the raspberry layer. Place the maple syrup and 2 tablespoons water in a saucepan and stir to combine over low heat. Bring to the boil and cook, without stirring, for 2–3 minutes or until the syrup thickens slightly. Remove from the heat and stir in the raspberries, then set aside to cool completely.

Place the raspberry mixture in a food processor and process until smooth. Strain through a fine sieve into a bowl, using a spatula to press as much pulp through as possible.

Gently spoon an even amount of the raspberry mixture over the yoghurt layer in each muffin mould. Cover and return to the freezer for another 2 hours or until set firm. Top with a little fresh mint to serve.

One yoghurt and raspberry sorbet is one serve. Leftovers may be covered and stored in the freezer for up to 2 months.

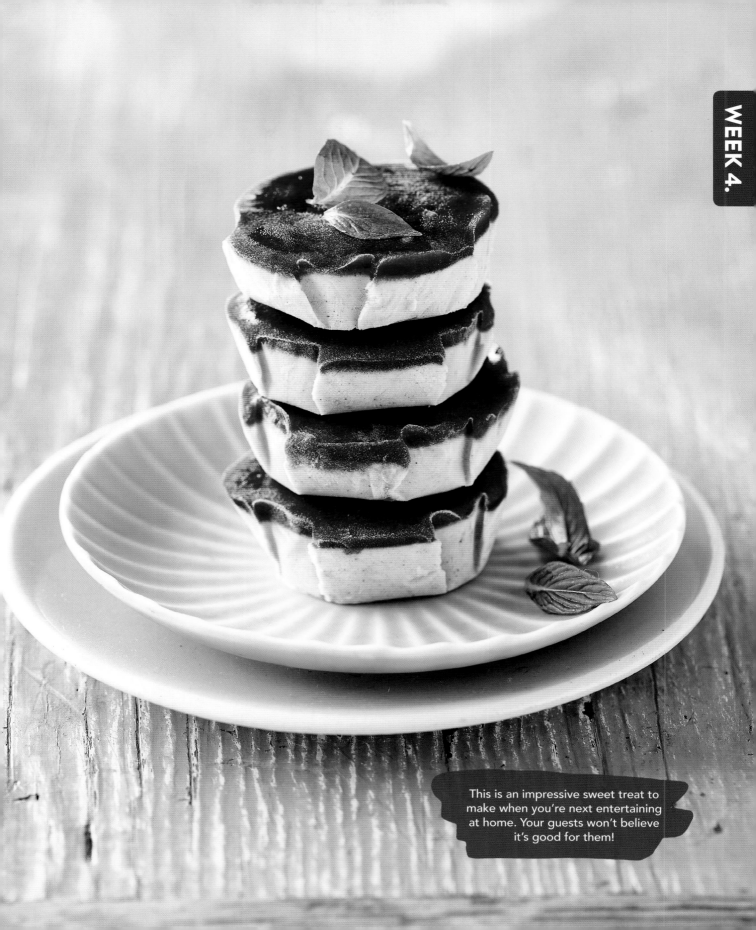

This is an impressive sweet treat to make when you're next entertaining at home. Your guests won't believe it's good for them!

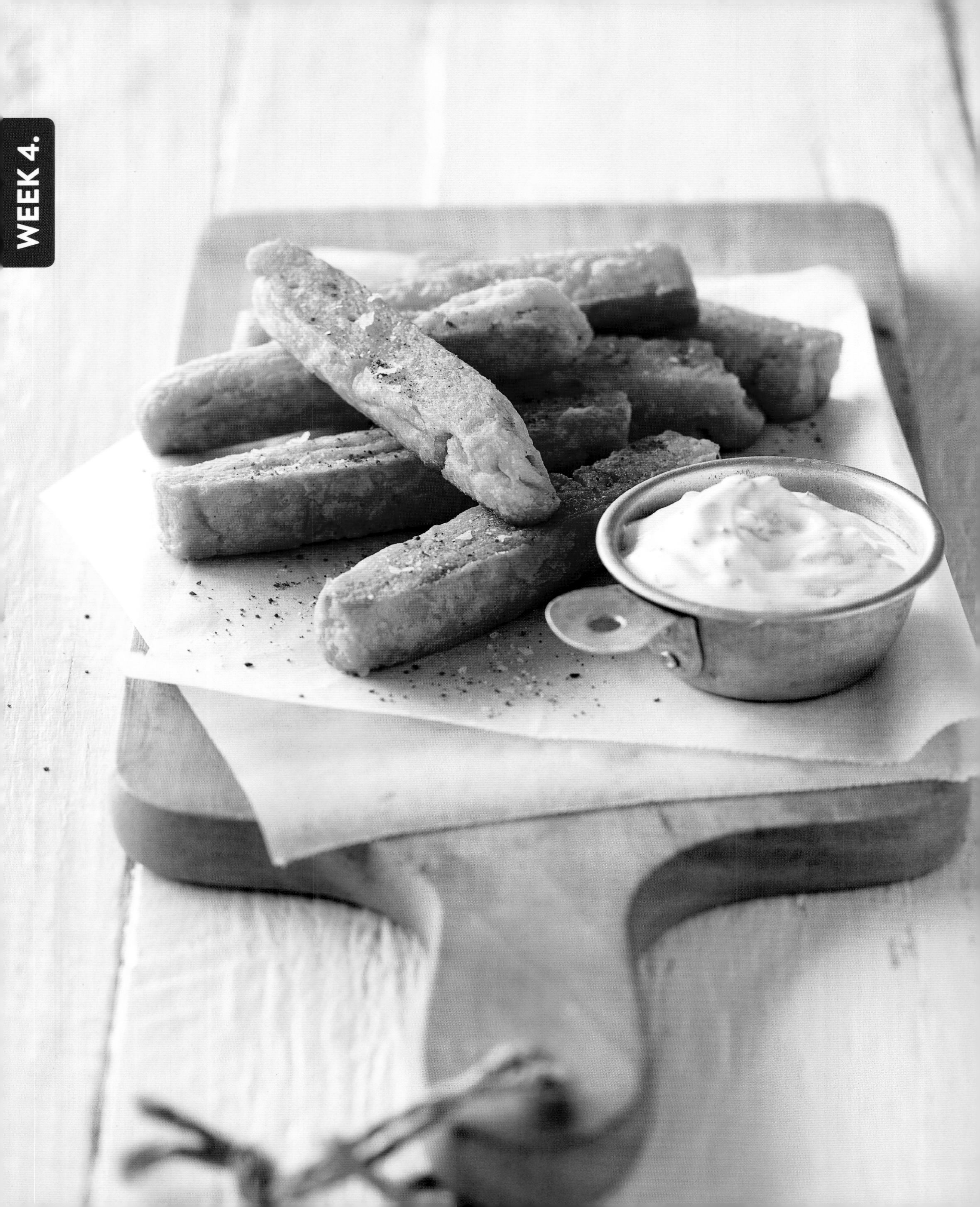

CHICKPEA FRIES WITH MINT SAUCE

SERVES: 1 **PREPARATION TIME:** 10 MINUTES, PLUS COOLING TIME **COOKING TIME:** 10 MINUTES

½ cup chickpea flour (besan)
¼ teaspoon ground cumin
salt
1 tablespoon coconut oil
¼ teaspoon ground sumac
2 tablespoons reduced-fat
  Greek-style yoghurt
5 mint leaves, finely chopped

NUTRI DETAILS PER SERVE

367 cals/1543 kjs
Protein: 12 g
Fibre: 5.2 g
Total fat: 22 g
Sat fat: 3 g
Carbs: 29.4 g
Total sugar: 8.1 g
Free sugar: 0.0 g

Place the chickpea flour, cumin, 150 ml water and a pinch of salt in a small saucepan and whisk until smooth. Place the pan over medium heat and cook, whisking constantly, for 2 minutes or until thickened.

Scrape the mixture onto a baking tray lined with baking paper and quickly smooth into a square or rectangle about 1 cm thick. Set aside to cool for 20 minutes or so, then cut into batons.

Heat the coconut oil in a frying pan over medium–high heat until it is hot (test by adding a small piece of the chickpea mixture to the pan – if it starts to form small bubbles and turns golden brown in 30 seconds, it's ready). Add the fries and cook, turning every minute or so, for 4 minutes or until golden brown on all sides. Drain on paper towel and sprinkle with the sumac and a little salt.

While the fries are cooking, mix together the yoghurt and mint to create the dipping sauce.

Serve the fries hot with the mint yoghurt.

SMOOTHIES

Mood-boosting smoothie

Almond chocolate
smoothie

Mint chocolate
sundae smoothie

MINT CHOCOLATE SUNDAE SMOOTHIE

SERVES: 1 **PREPARATION TIME:** 5 MINUTES

1 tablespoon rolled oats
2 tablespoons reduced-fat Greek-style yoghurt
2 teaspoons mint leaves
1 cup reduced-fat milk of choice
2 teaspoons cacao/cocoa powder
1 scoop vanilla soy ice-cream
1 teaspoon cacao nibs

Place the oats, yoghurt, mint, milk and cacao/cocoa powder in a blender and blitz until smooth. Scoop the ice-cream into a glass, pour the smoothie over the top and sprinkle with cacao nibs to serve.

NUTRI DETAILS PER SERVE

295 cals/1238 kjs	Sat fat: 4.6 g
Protein: 15.7 g	Carbs: 38 g
Fibre: 2 g	Total sugar: 25 g
Total fat: 8.5 g	Free sugar: 8 g

MOOD-BOOSTING SMOOTHIE

SERVES: 1 **PREPARATION TIME:** 5 MINUTES

1 banana
1 teaspoon cacao/cocoa powder
2 teaspoons chia seeds
200 ml soy milk
handful of ice cubes
5 walnuts
1 teaspoon spirulina powder

Place all the ingredients in a blender and blitz until smooth. Pour into a glass and serve.

NUTRI DETAILS PER SERVE

321 cals/1350 kjs	Sat fat: 2 g
Protein: 12.5 g	Carbs: 23.2 g
Fibre: 5.6 g	Total sugar: 15.3 g
Total fat: 19.5 g	Free sugar: 0.0 g

ALMOND CHOCOLATE SMOOTHIE

SERVES: 1 **PREPARATION TIME:** 5 MINUTES

1 tablespoon almond butter
¼ teaspoon ground cinnamon
½ banana
2 teaspoons cacao/cocoa powder
1 cup almond milk
½ teaspoon vanilla extract
¼ avocado

Place all the ingredients in a blender and blitz until smooth. Pour into a glass and serve.

NUTRI DETAILS PER SERVE

296 cals/1242 kjs	Sat fat: 3.4 g
Protein: 7.8 g	Carbs: 18.3 g
Fibre: 3.2 g	Total sugar: 10 g
Total fat: 22.5 g	Free sugar: 0.0 g

CHOCOLATE DOUGHNUT SMOOTHIE

SERVES: 1   **PREPARATION TIME:** 5 MINUTES

1 cereal wheat biscuit (such as Weet-Bix)
¾ cup reduced-fat milk of choice
2 teaspoons cacao/cocoa powder
3 tablespoons sunflower seeds
3 tablespoons reduced-fat coconut milk
1 teaspoon honey

Place all the ingredients in a blender and blitz until smooth. Pour into a glass and serve.

NUTRI DETAILS PER SERVE

287 cals/1204 kjs
Protein: 11.6 g
Fibre: 1.8 g
Total fat: 16.3 g

Sat fat: 13.2 g
Carbs: 23 g
Total sugar: 11.9 g
Free sugar: 0.0 g

THE BELLY BUSTER SMOOTHIE

SERVES: 1   **PREPARATION TIME:** 5 MINUTES

½ ruby red grapefruit, peeled
1 cup mixed berries (fresh or frozen)
3 tablespoons reduced-fat Greek-style yoghurt
1 tablespoon chia seeds
200 ml cold green tea
½ Lebanese cucumber, roughly chopped
1 ½ tablespoons raw almonds

Place all the ingredients in a blender and blitz until smooth. Pour into a glass and serve.

NUTRI DETAILS PER SERVE

294 cals/1236 kjs
Protein: 12.9 g
Fibre: 11 g
Total fat: 16.4 g

Sat fat: 1.9 g
Carbs: 21 g
Total sugar: 14 g
Free sugar: 0.0 g

BANANA BOOST SMOOTHIE

SERVES: 1   **PREPARATION TIME:** 5 MINUTES

200 ml reduced-fat milk of choice
½ frozen banana
3 tablespoons espresso
1 tablespoon oat bran
5 brazil nuts
1 teaspoon maca root powder
1 teaspoon pure maple syrup

Place all the ingredients in a blender and blitz until smooth. Pour into a glass and serve.

NUTRI DETAILS PER SERVE

344 cals/1444 kjs
Protein: 14.4 g
Fibre: 5.4 g
Total fat: 15.7 g

Sat fat: 4.6 g
Carbs: 35.5 g
Total sugar: 25.1 g
Free sugar: 4 g

Banana boost
smoothie

The
belly buster
smoothie

Chocolate doughnut
smoothie

FIBRE FULL SMOOTHIE

SERVES: 1   **PREPARATION TIME:** 5 MINUTES
PLUS SOAKING TIME

2 pitted dried dates
boiling water, for soaking
200 ml almond milk
½ banana
1 teaspoon psyllium husks
¼ teaspoon ground cinnamon
1 ½ tablespoons avocado
15 g kale leaves

Place the dates in a small heatproof bowl and
cover with boiling water. Leave to soak for
10 minutes, then drain.

Place all the ingredients in a blender and blitz
until smooth. Pour into a glass and serve.

NUTRI DETAILS PER SERVE

244 cals/1023 kjs	Sat fat: 1.3 g
Protein: 63 g	Carbs: 34 g
Fibre: 14.4 g	Total sugar: 28 g
Total fat: 8.5 g	Free sugar: 0.0 g

EXTRA ENERGY SMOOTHIE

SERVES: 1   **PREPARATION TIME:** 5 MINUTES

1 tablespoon chia seeds
½ cup reduced-fat coconut milk
1 teaspoon cacao/cocoa powder
3 tablespoons tinned black beans, drained and
   rinsed
1 teaspoon honey

Place all the ingredients and 1 cup water in a
blender and blitz until smooth. Pour into a glass
and serve.

NUTRI DETAILS PER SERVE

306 cals/1284 kjs	Sat fat: 19 g
Protein: 7.3 g	Carbs: 14.6 g
Fibre: 5.9 g	Total sugar: 3 g
Total fat: 24 g	Free sugar: 0.0 g

CHOCOLATE BANANA BREAD SMOOTHIE

SERVES: 1   **PREPARATION TIME:** 5 MINUTES

1 banana
2 teaspoons cacao/cocoa powder
¼ teaspoon ground cinnamon
¼ teaspoon vanilla extract
2 teaspoons cacao nibs
1 cup reduced-fat milk of choice
1 tablespoon quinoa flakes
1 teaspoon honey

Place all the ingredients in a blender and blitz
until smooth. Pour into a glass and serve.

NUTRI DETAILS PER SERVE

315 cals/1325 kjs	Sat fat: 4.7 g
Protein: 14 g	Carbs: 47.5 g
Fibre: 4.9 g	Total sugar: 34.9 g
Total fat: 7.6 g	Free sugar: 4 g

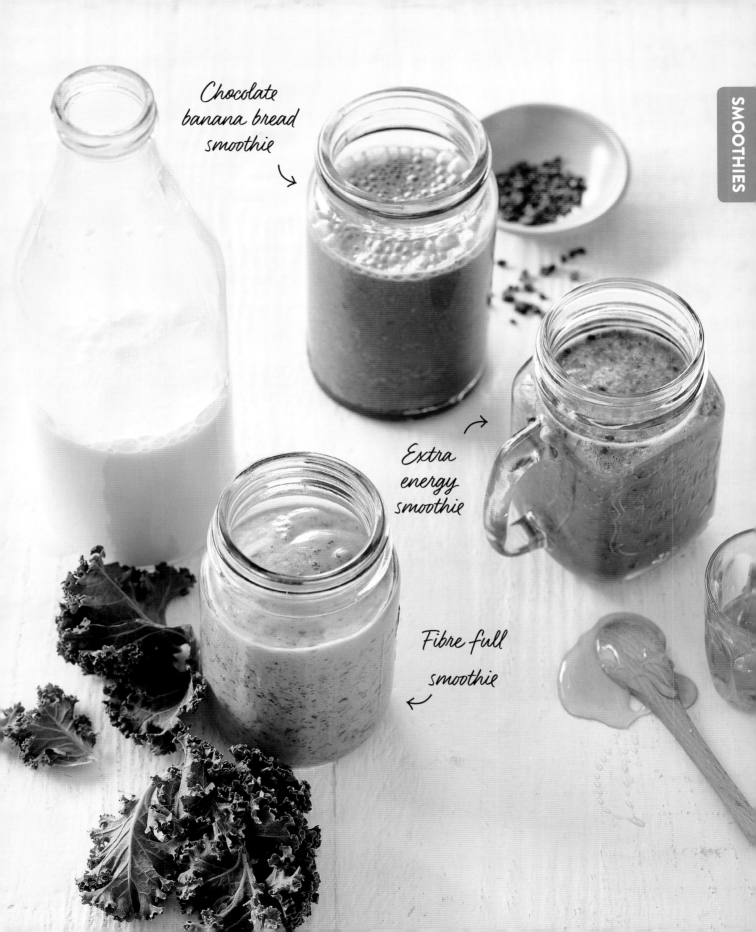

Chocolate
banana bread
smoothie

Extra
energy
smoothie

Fibre full
smoothie

ICED MOCHA SMOOTHIE

SERVES: 1   **PREPARATION TIME:** 5 MINUTES

1 teaspoon instant decaf coffee powder
½ cup boiling water
1 cup reduced-fat milk of choice
1 tablespoon cacao/cocoa powder
2 teaspoons cacao nibs
handful of ice cubes, plus extra to serve
1 ½ tablespoons unsalted cashews
1 teaspoon stevia

Dissolve the coffee powder in the boiling water. Place in a blender with the remaining ingredients and blitz until smooth. Pour into a glass, add extra ice if desired, and serve.

NUTRI DETAILS PER SERVE

296 cals/1243 kjs	Sat fat: 6.4 g
Protein: 15.6 g	Carbs: 21.4 g
Fibre: 3.5 g	Total sugar: 15 g
Total fat: 16.4 g	Free sugar: 0.0 g

THE BLOATED TUMMY SMOOTHIE

SERVES: 1   **PREPARATION TIME:** 5 MINUTES

1 teaspoon honey
½ banana
1 tablespoon mint leaves
3 tablespoons chopped papaya
3 tablespoons chopped pineapple
1 cup coconut water
3 tablespoons avocado
½ teaspoon chopped ginger
1 tablespoon reduced-fat Greek-style yoghurt

Place all the ingredients in a blender and blitz until smooth. Pour into a glass and serve.

NUTRI DETAILS PER SERVE

223 cals/ 932 kjs	Sat fat: 2.7 g
Protein: 5.1 g	Carbs: 26.7 g
Fibre: 3.7 g	Total sugar: 25 g
Total fat: 10 g	Free sugar: 4 g

APPLE PIE SMOOTHIE

SERVES: 1   **PREPARATION TIME:** 5 MINUTES

1 small apple, cored and roughly chopped
3 tablespoons rolled oats
½ teaspoon ground cinnamon
1 cup reduced-fat milk of choice
1 tablespoon low-fat cottage cheese

Place all the ingredients in a blender and blitz until smooth. Pour into a glass and serve.

NUTRI DETAILS PER SERVE

290 cals/1216 kjs	Sat fat: 2.8 g
Protein: 16 g	Carbs: 42 g
Fibre: 3.8 g	Total sugar: 26.6 g
Total fat: 6 g	Free sugar: 0.0 g

Iced mocha
smoothie
↓

The bloated
tummy smoothie
↓

Apple pie
smoothie

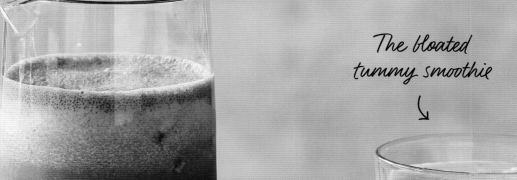

Vanilla blueberry smoothie

Date caramel smoothie

Sneaky 'snickers' smoothie

VANILLA BLUEBERRY SMOOTHIE

SERVES: 1   **PREPARATION TIME:** 5 MINUTES

½ banana
3 tablespoons blueberries (fresh or frozen)
2 teaspoons chia seeds
½ teaspoon ground cinnamon
1 cup reduced-fat milk of choice
1 teaspoon vanilla extract
3 tablespoons silken tofu
1 teaspoon honey

Place all the ingredients in a blender and blitz until smooth. Pour into a glass and serve.

NUTRI DETAILS PER SERVE

277 cals/ 1164 kjs	Sat fat: 3 g
Protein: 18 g	Carbs: 30.2 g
Fibre: 5.2 g	Total sugar: 25 g
Total fat: 9.5 g	Free sugar: 0.0 g

SNEAKY 'SNICKERS' SMOOTHIE

SERVES: 1   **PREPARATION TIME:** 5 MINUTES

1 banana
1 cup reduced-fat milk of choice
1 tablespoon peanut butter
3 tablespoons rolled oats
¼ teaspoon ground cinnamon, plus extra to sprinkle
1 teaspoon desiccated coconut

Place all the ingredients in a blender and blitz until smooth. Pour into a glass, sprinkle over extra cinnamon if desired, and serve.

NUTRI DETAILS PER SERVE

362 cals/1521 kjs	Sat fat: 4.8 g
Protein: 16.5 g	Carbs: 33.5 g
Fibre: 6 g	Total sugar: 23 g
Total fat: 17.4 g	Free sugar: 0.0 g

DATE CARAMEL SMOOTHIE

SERVES: 1   **PREPARATION TIME:** 5 MINUTES

3 tablespoons pitted dried dates
1 tablespoon unsalted cashews
¼ teaspoon vanilla extract
¼ teaspoon ground cinnamon
1 cup reduced-fat milk of choice
1 teaspoon tahini

Place all the ingredients in a blender and blitz until smooth. Pour into a glass and serve.

NUTRI DETAILS PER SERVE

350 cals/1472 kjs	Sat fat: 3.5 g
Protein: 13.7 g	Carbs: 47 g
Fibre: 5.8 g	Total sugar: 45 g
Total fat: 11.7 g	Free sugar: 0.0 g

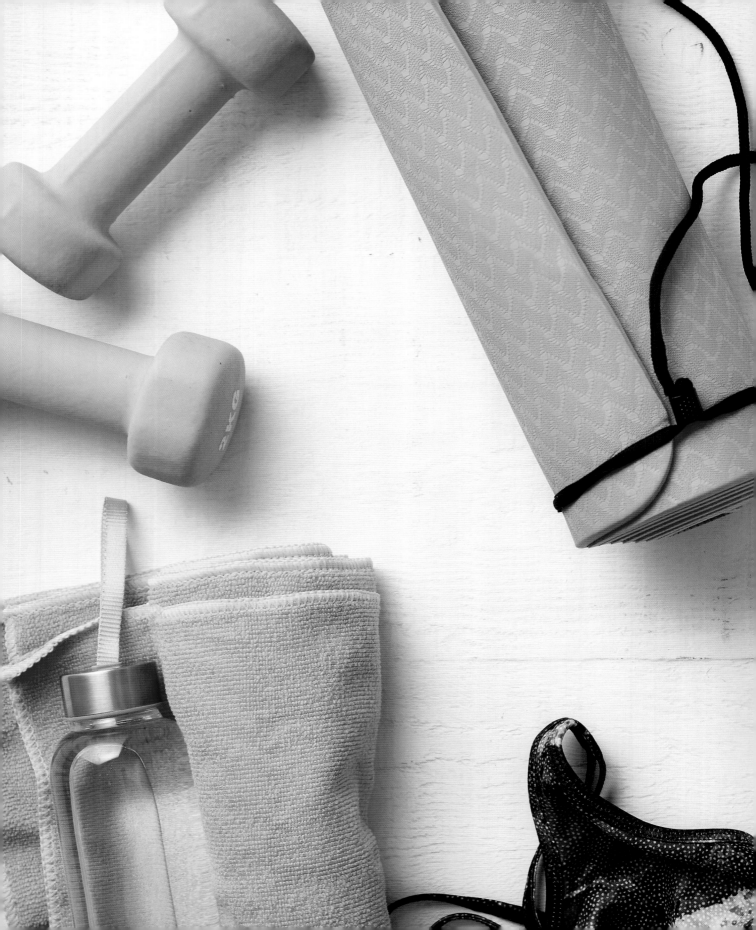

THE 28 DAY EXERCISE PLAN

Exercise is extremely important for physical health and mental wellbeing. The Healthy Mummy exercise plan is perfect for busy mums, as all the exercises can be done in the comfort of your own home. Refer to the meal and exercise plans at the start of each week, to see which workouts you need to do each day. And always remember to warm up and cool down at the start and end of each workout!

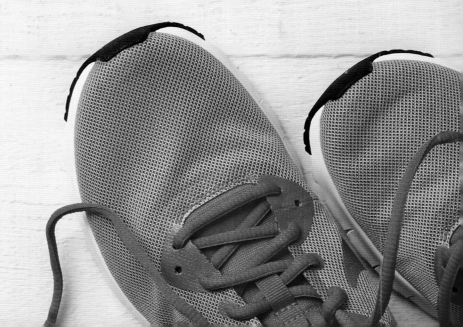

FINDING TIME TO EXERCISE

The main focus of the exercise plan is to simply try and increase your physical activity every day. In this section, we've outlined some short and snappy workouts that will help you burn calories in a short amount of time, as well as strengthen and tone your body all over – perfect for busy mums.

If you can't fit in the workouts each week as suggested, that's ok, just try and increase your physical activity as much as you can. This could be a short walk to the park with the kids, an easy jog around your neighbourhood, a few laps of the pool or just doing some squats and lunges while you're waiting for the kettle to boil!

Exercise is everywhere, and consciously deciding to move more will help you reach your weight-loss goals. Don't feel guilty if you miss a planned workout session, just try and fit something in when you can.

EXERCISING WITH A NEWBORN

The first few months of motherhood are exhausting and you'll most likely be feeling fatigued as you provide support for your new baby. You may be getting far less sleep than usual and your body is working hard to recover from the birth. It is, therefore, important to choose an exercise regime that feels right for you. If you are still in any pain or discomfort, take it easy and rest a little more before getting back into exercise. With a newborn, your life has to take on a new level of flexibility, and your exercise regime should, too.

If you're a mum with a newborn and following this plan, you may like to start slowly and perform each exercise on its own at different times. From there, you can work your way up to 3 sets of 5 minutes per day and then slowly increase these increments to 20 minutes or more per day. Even if you're only exercising for a few minutes at a time in those early stages, it all counts.

When your baby has settled more into a routine and you're feeling less tired, try scheduling your exercise time for just after you've fed your baby. This will be beneficial for you as you'll know when your workouts will be; it will also be far more comfortable for your body if you are breastfeeding. Plus your baby may even be asleep. Exercising while carrying your baby in a sling or pushing them in a pram is also a convenient way to exercise.

You may find you need to skip a day or two in the beginning to get a little more rest, and this is fine. Most importantly, you need to listen to your body, be gentle with yourself and take your time.

STRESS AND WEIGHT LOSS AFTER HAVING A BABY

When you're a new mum, lack of sleep and the pressure to get back to your 'pre-baby weight' are bound to cause stress. Recent studies suggest that managing stress is vital to weight loss and may even be more important than learning the specifics of nutrition and exercise. The stress hormone cortisol has a direct correlation with belly fat, and for many new mums that's the area they want to work on.

Fortunately, there are many ways you can reduce stress on both the body and mind. Going for a walk or meditating outside are excellent ways to give yourself some quiet reflection time and allow a change of scenery. Deep-breathing exercises are also great for reducing stress.

We're social creatures, so talking and spending time with others is another great way to feel supported during this time as a new mum. Try discussing your feelings and goals with your partner, a friend or family member. You may also like to join a postnatal exercise group as a way to keep fit and gain the support of other new mums who are in a similar situation.

FOUNDATIONS FIRST: YOUR CORE AND PELVIC FLOOR

The pelvic floor is imperative for bladder and bowel control. Without them, we would have limited (if any) control over our bladder and bowel movements. Eek!

In addition, the pelvic floor muscles work with the deep abdominal and back (core) muscles to help support and stabilise your spine.

It probably does not come as a surprise that your pelvic floor and core muscles are stretched (and weakened) during pregnancy and delivery. For this reason it is important to attend to these muscles before advancing with your exercise routine.

LOOKING AFTER YOUR PELVIC FLOOR FOR THE FUTURE

Did you know that one in three mothers suffers from incontinence? After having a baby, problems with bladder and bowel control can occur (as a result of weakened and stretched pelvic floor muscles). However, the good news is there is PLENTY you can do to improve their strength and decrease the risk of short- or long-term incontinence.

There is no doubt that specific exercises can help strengthen your pelvic floor, but it's important to recognise that not all exercises offer the same benefit. In fact, some exercises may cause you to overload the muscles and actually *lead* to incontinence, prolapse or back pain.

If you experience any of the following symptoms it may be a sign that you are overloading the pelvic floor. If this is the case, cease all exercise at once.

- Straining or bearing down
- Leakage/loss of control
- Heaviness or pressure
- Loss of awareness/inability to engage the muscles

TIPS FOR A HEALTHY PELVIC FLOOR

- Perform quality pelvic floor muscle-strengthening exercises 3 times a day.
- Avoid any exercise or activity that strains your pelvic floor.
- Activate your pelvic floor before lifting, exercise and actions such as laughing, sneezing and coughing.

KEEP YOUR BACK IN ACTION

From breastfeeding and changing nappies to hanging out the washing and popping your bub in the cot, there is no doubt a new mum's life includes many (many) activities that can put stress on your neck and upper back.

To avoid such aches and pains, be sure to do the following:

- Frequently lengthen your spine and roll your shoulders up, back and down.
- Check your posture regularly and avoid rounding your neck and back, especially when feeding.
- Include neck and shoulder mobility, upper-back strengthening and stretches that elongate the muscles at the front of your chest and shoulders to combat any tendency to slouch.

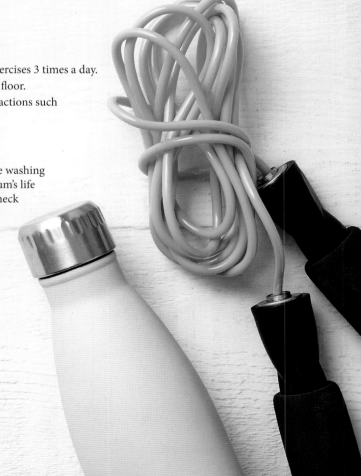

GENERAL TIPS FOR MUMS GETTING BACK INTO EXERCISE

- Prioritise your core and pelvic floor.
- Listen to your body.
- Include rest and relaxation as part of your overall wellbeing plan.
- Enjoy a healthy, balanced diet, full of lean proteins, fruits and vegetables, and avoid junk foods.
- Drink plenty of water.
- Get out and about: fresh air is great for your body and your soul.
- Wear comfortable clothing and good, underwire-free breast support.
- Rest up if you feel exhausted or unwell and never exercise in the presence of fever.
- Be kind to yourself and be patient.

HOW MUCH IS TOO MUCH?

Listen to your body. This guide will help you determine whether you are at the right level.

- You should be able to talk throughout your workout.
- Check that your movement is consistently smooth and controlled.
- Holding your breath, straining, shaking or tensing other muscles (such as shrugging your shoulders) are all signs that you are overdoing it.

If you experience any signs of lightheadedness, bleeding and/or shakiness during or after exercise, it is important that you stop your workout and organise a chat with your healthcare professional.

DOMS

When you start a new exercise routine you'll be asking your muscles to work a little harder than they might be used to, and there is a chance you may experience delayed-onset muscle soreness (DOMS). But don't worry, this is incredibly common – especially if you haven't worked a certain muscle group in a while.

The thing about DOMS is that you don't necessarily feel soreness straight after training; it may take 24–48 hours to kick in (hence 'delayed-onset'). What's more, you may not be aware of the soreness at rest, but as soon as you start to move around you can feel it.

It's important to understand that DOMS IS NOT AN INJURY and does not require medical attention. The only thing you can do is let it subside in its own time, and this can take up to 7 days.

The best way to prevent DOMS is to ease yourself into a new exercise routine, letting your muscles get used to new movements before putting them under too much strain. After a couple of weeks, your muscles will be ready to increase the intensity of the exercise and you will be far less likely to experience DOMS.

POSTNATAL EXERCISE

THE FIRST FEW WEEKS

The first couple of weeks after having a baby should be a time for rest, so pop those feet up when you can and let your body recover. It's very important that your energy levels increase naturally and you allow your pelvic floor and perineum to recover. This is certainly not the time to work out vigorously.

Performing simple pelvic floor and core exercises three times a day and walking within your comfort zone is all the exercise you need to think about at this stage.

GUIDELINES

It is really important that you talk to your obstetrician, medical doctor, midwife and/or physiotherapist prior to starting an exercise regime following birth.

The basic guidelines below will help you move towards commencing the postnatal workouts outlined in the plan.

1. It is generally recommended that you wait until your 6-week postnatal doctor's appointment prior to starting the workouts. That way, your doctor can suggest exercises that are safe for you to start with.

2. You may decide to do some abdominal muscle and pelvic floor testing before commencing any new workouts (see Abdominal Separation on the next page for further details). If you are suffering from abdominal separation or recovering from a C-section or prolapse, there are specific exercises that can help with your recovery.

3. About 12 weeks after birth, your doctor may advise that it is safe to gradually increase the intensity of your workouts. For example, it may be safe to start some light walking.

4. Exercises such as Leg Lifts, V Lifts, Planks and Mountain Climbers, which put pressure on the abdominals and mid-section, are not usually recommended and should not be tried until those muscles have reached full strength.

5. If you are recovering from a C-section, prolapse, abdominal separation or are simply unsure of your circumstances, check with your health professional first and always protect your body by choosing the low-impact versions of the workouts provided in the plan.

6. Between 16 and 20 weeks after birth, your body is generally ready to return to its previous activities, providing your pelvic floor and abdominals have regained their strength and you are not experiencing any pain or bleeding. Of course, always check with your healthcare professionals prior to beginning any exercise regime.

There is no doubt that postnatal exercise has incredible physical and mental benefits. However, exercising too soon can lead to serious injury. It is important that you let your body recover post birth and work out wisely and with great care.

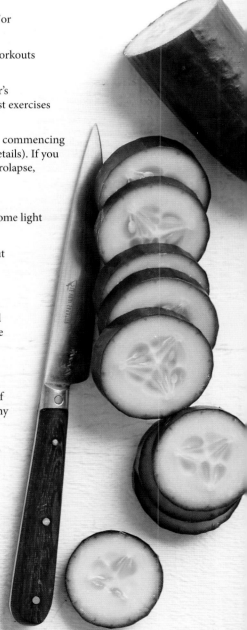

BDOMINAL SEPARATION

you have separated abs? If you have been pregnant several times, you're more likely to have diastasis recti, or separated abdominal muscles. This is because the muscles stretch every time you are pregnant and, like a stretched rubber band, cracks are more likely to develop. Exercising throughout pregnancy is a good way to avoid this condition.

If you haven't been checked for diastasis recti by your healthcare professional, here's a guide to examining yourself:

STEP 1

Lie down with your knees bent and place your right hand behind your head.

STEP 2

With your left hand, put your index and middle fingers together and place them horizontally in the centreline of your stomach between your abdominals.

STEP 3

From here, slowly raise your head slightly off the floor, while supporting it with your right hand. Don't just lift your head with your hand – lift through your pelvic floor and transverse abdominal muscle to gently lift your shoulders off the floor and feel the abdominals to get the best assessment of your separation.

STEP 4

By now, your abdominals will be contracting slightly and you will feel exactly how far your abdominals have separated.

STEP 5

If the index and middle fingers on your left hand can still fit between your abdominals you have diastasis recti of 2–2.5 cm. For every additional finger you can place between your abdominals add 1 cm to your total abdominal separation number. If you can only fit one finger between your abdominals you effectively have 1 cm of separation and are nearly healed.

If there is more than 1 cm separation you should refrain from doing exercises, such as crunches, sit-ups or pilates 'hundreds' as all of these can put too much pressure on the abdominal muscles separated during pregnancy and potentially cause further damage to the muscles and ligaments.

If you do have muscle separation, PLEASE see a physio before starting any exercise. They will examine you and confirm the level of your separation; in addition, they will advise you on the level of gentle exercise to do and when you will be ready to begin.

EXERCISES TO DO AFTER A CAESAREAN

While caesarean techniques can vary, they all involve a surgical procedure and the opening of the lower abdominal wall. This means you need to take extra care when you're recovering and returning to exercise.

While you're in the early stages of recovering from a C-section, you will benefit from performing some very simple exercises 3 times a day:

- **Pelvic floor exercises:** 3 long lifts or 5–8 quick lifts will help strengthen your pelvic floor and assist in preventing incontinence and other problems later on.

- **Core strengthening:** Your deepest abdominal and back muscles support the spine and pelvis, and provide foundation strength for all other activities. As soon as it's comfortable for you, you can slowly start to regain their strength and control. Gently draw your lower abdomen inwards and upwards and hold for 3–5 breaths. Relax and repeat for 3 more rounds. Make sure you are breathing normally and that you are not sucking in your waist or ribs as you draw in below the navel.

- **Easy foot and leg movements:** Next time you're resting in bed, try waving your feet back and forth 10 times and bending and straightening your knees 5 times on each leg. This will help maintain healthy blood flow.

- **Gentle neck and shoulder movements:** These will help to minimise stiffness in the neck and shoulder area and are particularly helpful for mums with post-caesarean postural problems. Sit up tall to lengthen your spine, then roll your shoulders slowly up, back and down 10 times. Then, carefully roll your head and neck in a small circle 3 times in each direction.

As time passes, continue your pelvic floor exercises and neck and shoulder stretches. When you combine these with getting up and looking after your new bub, you'll be getting enough exercise. However, you should avoid any heavy lifting or strenuous activity for at least 6 weeks.

When you are comfortable, you can start taking some light walks. Getting out and about with your baby in the pram is not only great for your body, it's also great for your mental health. Begin with a 5-minute stroll and gradually increase your time, monitoring your comfort and energy levels.

WHAT NOT TO DO:

- Too much, too soon.
- Put too much stress or expectation on your body (scar included) or mind.
- Lift anything heavier than your baby for 6–12 weeks.
- Exercise if you feel unwell or tired or have any pain or concern.
- Exercise in the water until there is no more lochia (vaginal discharge post caesarean) and your incision is well healed.
- Any exercise where you can't maintain your pelvic floor and engage your core throughout.

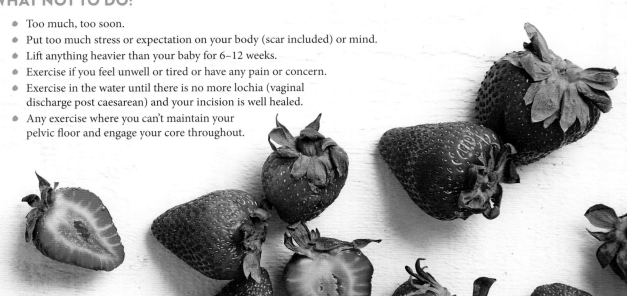

THE
WORKOUTS

WARM UP

Warming up is an essential part of any workout as it prepares your body for exercise by loosening up the muscles, ligaments and joints. A short warm up of 3–5 minutes using simple, easy-to-perform exercises will have your body ready to start your workout.

When starting the 28 day plan, complete the warm-up exercises below for 3–5 minutes before starting your daily workouts. At the end of your workout complete the cool-down exercises on pages 306–307.

ABDOMINAL BREATHING

Sit up straight and focus your breath in your belly, expanding as you inhale and contracting as you exhale. Place your hands on your belly so you can feel the in-breath and out-breath.

JOG ON THE SPOT

Keep good posture with your head up, shoulders back and core engaged as you gently jog on the spot.

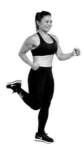

BREATHING

When performing weight-bearing exercise, it's important to ensure that your breathing remains steady. By breathing correctly during exercise your body and brain gets all the oxygen it needs, avoiding light-headedness and early fatigue. It can be tempting to hold your breath when exerting force during an exercise (e.g. lifting, pushing, pulling etc.). Using the squat as an example, we recommend breathing in on the way down and exhaling as you push back up.

STARTING POSITIONS

Many of our exercises begin in one of the following starting positions.

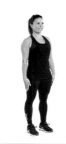

STANDING

Stand with your feet shoulder-width apart with your arms by your sides. Keep your head facing forward, relax your shoulders and gently engage your core.

PUSH UP ON KNEES

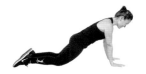

Start in an all-fours position. Walk your hands forward until your body is in a straight line from your shoulders to your knees. Keep your hands directly under your shoulders. Try not to hunch your shoulders. Keep your eyes focused on the floor between your hands.

PLANK (ON HANDS OR ELBOWS)

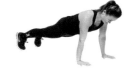

Start in an all-fours position on hands or elbows. Push up onto your toes. Keep your hands or elbows directly under your shoulders and engage your core to make sure your body is in a straight line without sagging in the middle. Keep your eyes focused on the floor between your hands.

LAYING ON BACK

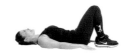

Lay on your back with your knees bent and your feet flat on the floor. Your spine should have two areas that do not touch the mat underneath you: your neck and your lower back. It's important to maintain the natural curves in your spine to prevent lower back and neck strain. Some exercises will then ask you to press your spine into the mat, but it's good to start in this neutral position.

LAYING ON BACK WITH LEGS IN TABLE-TOP POSITION

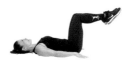

Begin by laying on your back as above. Keep your arms on the floor beside you. Draw your knees up so your shins are straight (like a table-top). Draw your belly button towards the floor to engage your core.

16 MINUTE TUMMY TAMER WORKOUTS

These are the perfect workouts to strengthen your core. They are made up of functional exercises that mimic everyday movements like twisting, balancing, pushing and reaching.

Focus on keeping your core engaged during the active phase of each movement. Draw your belly button in towards your spine and imagine you are not only contracting your stomach muscles vertically, but also horizontally around, like pulling in a belt.

WORKOUT 1

Perform each exercise for 1 minute with a 10 second rest between exercises. Complete the entire circuit 4 times.

1. BURPEE WITH LEG LIFT

Place your hands on the floor in front of you, jump your feet out to plank position, then jump them back in and return to standing. Take a big jump, lifting your arms above your head, then lift one leg out to the side. Repeat the exercise on the other side.

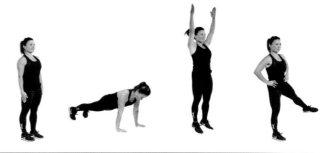

2. PIKE WALK WITH PUSH UP

Place your hands on the floor in front of you and walk them out until you are in plank position. Do a push up. Bend your knees slightly, walk your hands back in and come to standing.

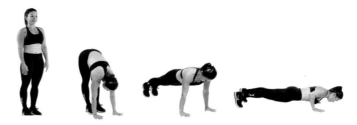

3. LUNGE WITH TWIST

Take a big long step forward, dropping the back knee close to the ground. Rotate your upper body to the right then twist back to lunge position. Push off your front foot to a standing position. Alternate legs and repeat.

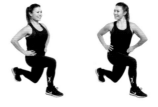

4. PLANK WITH KNEE DRIVE

Start in a plank on elbows position and, keeping your body in a straight line, alternate bringing your knees in towards the opposite elbow.

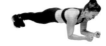 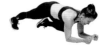

WORKOUT 2

**Perform each exercise for 1 minute with a 10 second rest between exercises.
Complete the entire circuit 4 times.**

1. **OVERHEAD BALL THROW**

Keep your knees soft and bouncy, and take
a shallow squat between each throw.

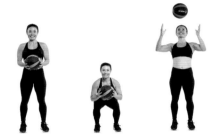

2. **V-LIFT WITH OBLIQUE TWIST**

Keep your legs straight up, hold the ball
overhead and lift your shoulders off the floor
as you reach the ball past your legs on one side.
Return to the start position and repeat on
the other side.

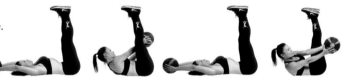

3. **STANDING OBLIQUE CRUNCH**

With your feet together, lower into a squat
and, as you come back to standing, lift one leg
out and up towards your armpit. Return to
standing and repeat on the other side.

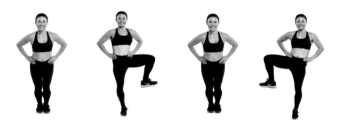

4. **BENT KNEE PUSH UP**

Keeping your back straight, bend your elbows
until your chest is about 7-8 cm from the floor.
Pause and push back to starting position.

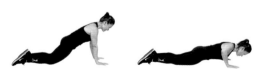

LOW IMPACT 20 MINUTE TUMMY TAMER WORKOUT

The low impact variation of the 16 minute tummy tamer workout is suitable for women recovering from a C-section or those with abdominal separation and/or a weak pelvic floor.

LOW IMPACT VARIATION

Perform each exercise for 1 minute with a 10 second rest between exercises. Complete the entire circuit 4 times.

1. TOE TAPS

Start on your back with legs in table-top position. Engage your core and tap your toes on the floor using a slow and controlled movement, alternating left and right.

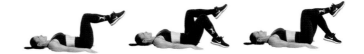

2. FOUR POINT KNEELING

Start on all fours and raise one arm out in front of you and the opposite leg out behind you, then bring them back to the floor. Repeat on the other side. If you find this exercise difficult, you don't need to lift the arm and leg at the same time. This will still be effective lifting one limb at a time.

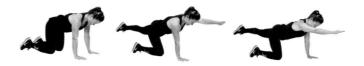

3. WINDSHIELD WIPER

Start in table-top position. Using a controlled movement, lower both legs to one side. Return them to the centre and repeat on the other side. Keep your core engaged.

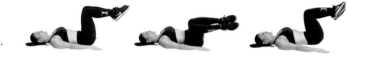

4. PELVIC TILT WITH MODIFIED BRIDGE

Contract your pelvic floor muscles and imagine moving your pubic bone towards your belly button. To finish the exercise, push through your heels and lift your hips off the floor, squeezing your glutes.

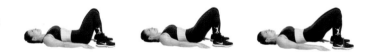

5. BRIDGE WITH DUMBBELL FLY

Lift your hips off the floor and bring the dumbbells together in front of you. With palms facing in, lower the dumbbells to the sides, level with your chest and repeat.

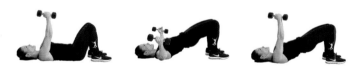

20 MINUTE
METABOLIC BOOSTER WORKOUTS

The aim of the metabolic booster workouts is to get your heart pumping, using a combination of cardio and strength exercises that work your whole body. When you increase your muscle mass, you boost your resting metabolism, and that makes your body burn more calories!

WORKOUT 1

Perform each exercise for 1 minute with a 10 second rest between exercises.
Complete the entire circuit 4 times.

1. HIGH SKIP

Using an imaginary rope, lift your knees high and maintain good posture as you skip on the spot.

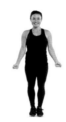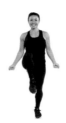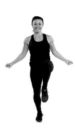

2. MOUNTAIN CLIMBER

Start in plank position and alternate bringing each knee in towards your chest. Focus on keeping your body in a straight line.

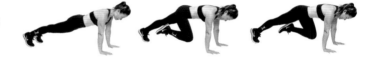

3. JUMP TOUCHDOWN

Start with your arms up above your head. Lower into a deep squat and touch the floor before jumping up and beginning again.

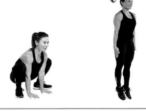

4. BICYCLE

Focus on keeping your core very stable as you cycle your legs. Do this by drawing your navel in towards your spine.

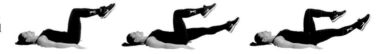

5. DANCING JACKS

Jump your legs out and raise your arms in front, then jump back in. Jump your legs out again, but this time raise your arms out to the sides. Repeat.

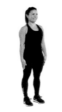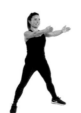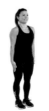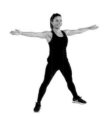

WORKOUT 2

Perform each exercise for 1 minute with a 10 second rest between exercises.
Complete the entire circuit 4 times.

1. OVERHEAD JACKS

Keep your torso in alignment as you jump your legs out and raise your arms out to the side.

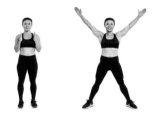

2. DUMBBELL STEP UP

Hold the dumbbells at your sides. Step up and down on one side for 30 seconds before swapping legs.

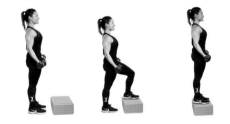

3. BICYCLE

Keep your core stable as you cycle your legs. Do this by drawing your navel in towards your spine.

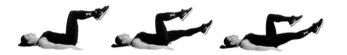

4. BURPEE WITH LEG LIFT

Place your hands on the floor in front of you, jump your feet out to plank position, then jump them back in and return to standing. Take a big jump, lifting your arms above your head, then lift one leg out to the side. Repeat the exercise on the other side.

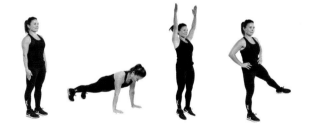

5. SINGLE HIGH JUMP

Bend into a deep squat and jump as high as you can. Tuck your feet right up when you jump and land gently on both feet.

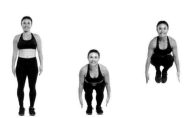

20 MINUTE BODY STRONG PILATES WORKOUTS

These Pilates workouts are designed to build muscle endurance and burn calories. When performing each exercise, keep your movements slow and controlled so your muscles receive the maximum benefit. During a Pilates workout it is not about how many repetitions you complete, but about ensuring that you maintain good technique for the duration of the exercise.

WORKOUT 1
Complete the entire circuit twice – 1 minute per exercise.

1. PILATES LEG CIRCLE

Lay on your back and stretch one leg towards the ceiling. Sweep it around in large circles, keeping your pelvis and shoulders on the floor. Repeat with the other leg.

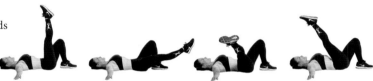

2. PILATES HIP LIFTS

Place a ball between your knees and squeeze it as you come into a bridge. Pump the pelvis up and down and don't drop the ball!

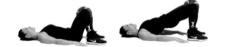

3. PILATES BRIDGE POSE KNEE LIFT

Come into bridge position and raise one knee towards your chest. Repeat with the other leg. Remember to keep your core engaged.

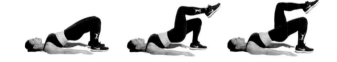

4. PILATES SIDE SCISSORS

Lay on your side, with your head resting on your arm. Place your other hand on the floor in front of you. With your feet together, lift them slightly off the floor and kick them backwards and forwards like scissors.

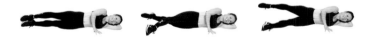

5. PILATES MERMAID WITH WAIST STRETCH

Sit in a side seat with your left hand on the floor. Reach your right arm over your head and stretch over, then reach under your arm. Repeat on the other side.

6. FIRE HYDRANT

Start on all fours. Lift one leg out to the side, then repeat on the other side. Keep your neck and spine in good alignment.

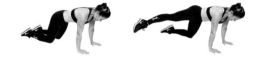

7. PILATES TRICEP PUSH UP

Start on all fours. Bring your hands together on the floor in front of you. Spread your fingers, bend through your elbows and lower your chest towards the floor. Push up to starting position.

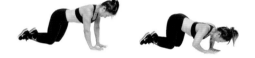

8. PILATES PLIÉ PULSES

Start in standing position with your feet turned out. Keep your back upright and lower down into a squat position, keeping your knees in line with your feet. Pulse up and down gently.

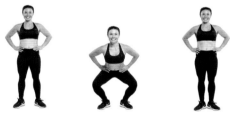

9. PILATES STAND AND SWIM

Come into a squat and raise your arms out in front of you. Paddle your arms with small up and down movements.

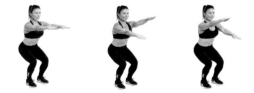

10. PILATES ROLL DOWN

Start with your arms stretched above you. Exhale, tuck your chin in and roll down slowly. Inhale and roll up slowly, finishing with your arms in the starting position.

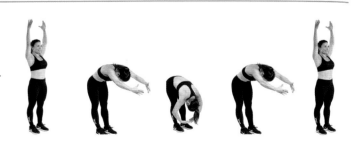

20 MINUTE BODY STRONG PILATES WORKOUTS

WORKOUT 2

Complete the entire circuit twice – 1 minute per exercise.

1. PILATES HIP LIFTS

Place a ball between your knees and squeeze it as you come into a bridge. Pump the pelvis up and down and don't drop the ball!

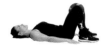 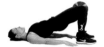

2. ROPE CLIMB

Lean your body back until you feel your core engage, then hold an imaginary rope and pretend to climb.

  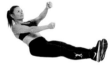

3. PILATES TRICEP PUSH UP

Start on all fours. Bring your hands together on the floor in front of you. Spread your fingers, bend through your elbows and lower your chest towards the floor. Push up to starting position.

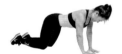 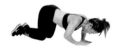

4. PILATES ABDOMINAL SWING

Start in table-top position with your hands behind your knees, then inhale. Exhale as you straighten your legs, point your toes, lift your upper body and roll forward slightly.

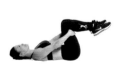

5. PILATES TOE TAPS

Start on your back with legs in table-top position. Engage your core and tap your toes on the floor, alternating left and right.

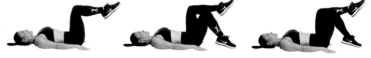

6. PILATES INNER THIGH LIFT

Lie on the floor on your right side with your legs straight. Exhale, engage your core and scissor your legs apart. Lift your left leg and hold. Keeping your leg straight, inhale and slowly lift your right leg in line with your left leg. Exhale and return your legs to the floor. Alternate sides.

7. PILATES DOUBLE LEG LIFT

Lie on the floor on your right side with your legs straight. Engage your core and lift both legs off the floor. Slowly lift your left leg away from your right leg. Return your left leg to meet your right leg. Alternate sides.

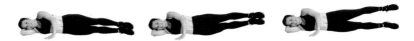

8. PILATES FLYING WINGS

Stand in an upright position with your legs wide and feet turned out. Bend your knees and sit down into a squat position. Inhale as you lift your arms out in front of you to shoulder height, engage your core and push back up to standing position.

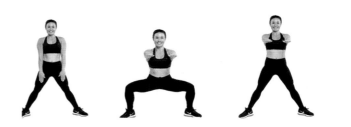

9. PILATES STAND AND SWIM

Come into a squat and raise your arms out in front of you. Paddle your arms with small up and down movements.

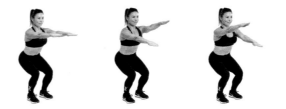

10. PILATES ROLL DOWN

Start with your arms stretched above you. Exhale, tuck your chin in and roll down slowly. Inhale and roll up slowly, finishing with your arms in the starting position.

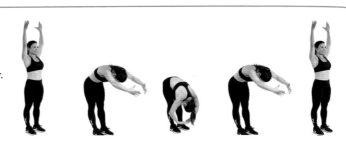

20 MINUTE DEEP CORE CONDITIONING WORKOUTS

The 'core' is a term used to describe the glutes, hips, abdominal muscles, pelvic floor and back. A strong core provides a firm foundation for exercise, helping to prevent injury, and allowing you to perform any movement with stability. Training your core is not complicated, but it is important to focus on good technique.

WORKOUT 1

Perform each exercise for 1 minute with a 10 second rest between exercises. Complete the entire circuit 4 times.

1. SIDE STEP UP

Focus on keeping the movement slow and controlled. Bring one foot onto the step and bring the other foot up to meet it. Step down and repeat. Alternate sides on each round.

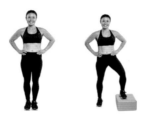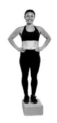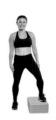

2. BICYCLE WITH BALL PASS

Focus on keeping your core engaged and use controlled movements as you pass the ball under your legs.

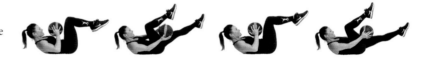

3. V-LIFT WITH OBLIQUE TWIST

Keep your legs straight up, hold the ball overhead and lift your shoulders off the floor as you reach the ball past your legs on one side. Return to the start position and repeat on the other side.

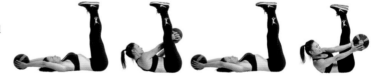

4. PIKE WALK WITH PUSH UP

Place your hands on the floor in front of you and walk them out until you are in plank position. Do a push up. Bend your knees slightly, walk your hands back in and come to standing.

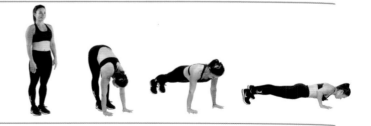

5. KNEE SIDE PLANK WITH ARM RAISE

Lay on your left side, with the knee closest to the floor bent at a 90 degree angle. Support yourself on your left elbow, keeping the elbow directly below your shoulder. Engage your glutes and lift your hips off the floor. Extend your right arm towards the roof and slowly return your hip to the floor. Repeat on the other side.

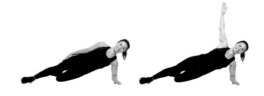

WORKOUT 2

Perform each exercise for 1 minute with a 10 second rest between exercises. Complete the entire circuit 4 times.

1. ROPE CLIMB

Lean your body back until you feel your core engage, then hold an imaginary rope and pretend to climb.

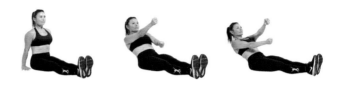

2. BRIDGE WITH BALL

Place a ball between your knees and squeeze it as you come into a bridge. Come up onto your toes and don't drop the ball!

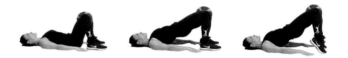

3. ROTATIONAL SIDE PLANK

Focus on keeping your side plank straight. Keep your shoulders stable and use a controlled movement to reach your top arm down and through.

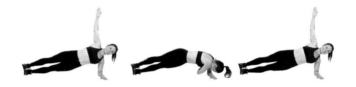

4. MOVING REVERSE BRIDGE

Focus on contracting your core and glutes to form a straight line between your shoulders and ankles. Use a controlled movement to swing your hips back between your hands, keeping your hips off the floor.

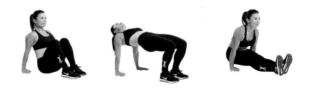

5. KNEE SIDE PLANK WITH ARM RAISE

Lay on your left side, with the knee closest to the floor bent at a 90 degree angle. Support yourself on your left elbow, keeping the elbow directly below your shoulder. Engage your glutes and lift your hips off the floor. Extend your right arm towards the roof and slowly return your hip to the floor. Repeat on the other side.

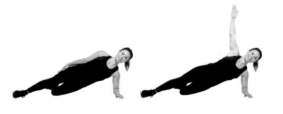

LOW IMPACT 20 MINUTE DEEP CORE CONDITIONING WORKOUT

The low impact variation of the deep core conditioning workout is suitable for women recovering from a C-section or those with abdominal separation and/or a weak pelvic floor.

LOW IMPACT VARIATION

Perform each exercise for 1 minute with a 10 second rest between exercises. Complete the entire circuit 4 times.

1. TOE TAPS

Start on your back with legs in table-top position. Engage your core and tap your toes on the floor using a slow and controlled movement, alternating left and right.

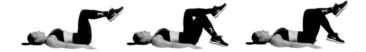

2. BICYCLE

Keep your core stable as you cycle your legs. Do this by drawing your navel in towards your spine.

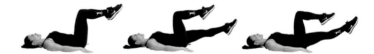

3. SINGLE LEG LIFT

Keep one leg extended and slightly off the floor.
Keeping your other leg straight, raise it towards
you before lowering it back down to meet
the other leg. Repeat for 30 seconds before
switching legs.

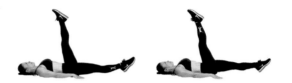

4. ALPHABET LEG CIRCLE

Write the alphabet with your extended leg.
Remember to engage your core and keep your
pelvis stable. Repeat with the other leg.

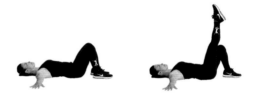

5. FOUR POINT KNEELING

Start on all fours and raise one arm out
in front of you and the opposite leg
out behind you, then bring them back
to the floor. Repeat on the other side.
If you find this exercise difficult, you
don't need to lift the arm and leg at the
same time. Lifting one limb at a time
will still be effective.

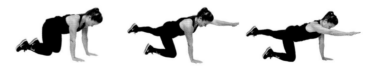

LOW IMPACT 12 MINUTE TOTAL BODY TABATA WORKOUT

The low impact variation of the Total Body Tabata workout is suitable for women recovering from a C-section or those with abdominal separation and/or a weak pelvic floor.

LOW IMPACT VARIATION

Perform each exercise for 1 minute with a 10 second rest between exercises.
Complete the entire circuit 2 times.

1. **MID SQUAT WITH FORWARD JAB**

Keep your stance wide and deep with your toes pointing outwards. Engage your core and punch with power!

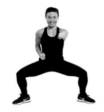 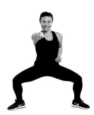

2. **KNEE SIDE PLANK WITH ARM RAISE**

Lay on your left side, with the knee closest to the floor bent at a 90 degree angle. Support yourself on your left elbow, keeping the elbow directly below your shoulder. Engage your glutes and lift your hips off the floor. Extend your right arm towards the roof and slowly return your hip to the floor. Repeat on the other side.

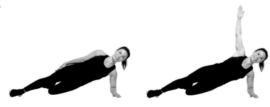

3. **BENT KNEE PUSH UP**

Keeping your back straight, bend your elbows until your chest is about 7–8 cm from the floor. Pause and push back to starting position.

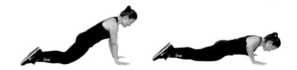

4. LUNGE PULSES

Take a big, long step forward, dropping the back knee close to the ground and pulse up and down. To avoid injury, make sure your front knee does not extend beyond your toe. Pump on one leg for one round and then alternate legs for the next round.

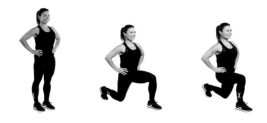

5. SQUAT PUMPS

Keep your attention on your core as you sink down into a squat position. Ensure your knees don't go past your toes and keep your back straight and shoulders back. Lift your arms in front of you and hold the squat position for 1–2 seconds, then gently pump up and down before returning to start position.

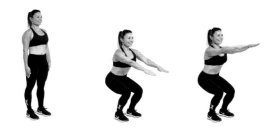

6. LOW IMPACT JACKS

Keep your torso in alignment and raise your arms out to the sides, as you step your legs out. Lower into a squat, then return to standing.

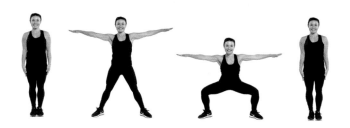

14 MINUTE TOTAL BODY TABATA WORKOUT

'Tabata' is high-intensity interval training inspired by Dr Izumi Tabata, a Japanese researcher who found that all-out extreme intensity exercise for a short period, followed by 10 seconds of rest, improved both the aerobic and anaerobic systems of the athletes he studied.

> **Perform each exercise for 1 minute with a 10 second rest between exercises. Complete the entire circuit 2 times.**

1. OVERHEAD JACKS

Keep your torso in alignment as you jump your legs out and raise your arms out to the side.

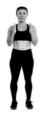 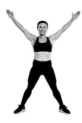

2. SQUAT PUMPS

Keep your attention on your core as you sink down into a squat position. Ensure your knees don't go past your toes and keep your back straight and shoulders back. Lift your arms in front of you and hold the squat position for 1–2 seconds, then gently pump up and down before returning to start position.

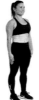 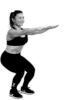

3. HIGH SKIP

Using an imaginary rope, lift your knees high and maintain good posture as you skip on the spot.

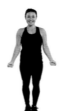 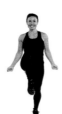 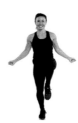

4. MOUNTAIN CLIMBER

Start in plank position and alternate bringing each knee in towards your chest. Focus on keeping your body in a straight line.

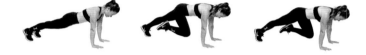

5. LOW IMPACT JACKS

Keep your torso in alignment and raise your arms out to the sides, as you step your legs out. Lower into a squat, then return to standing.

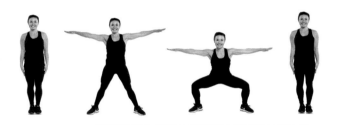

6. ON-THE-SPOT SPRINT

Run as fast as you can on the spot.

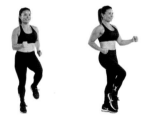

7. ELBOW PLANK WITH SIDE WALK

Start in plank position on your elbows and step both of your feet to one side, then the other. Keep your body in a straight line.

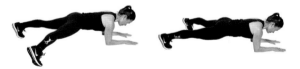

20 MINUTE BUTT AND THIGH WORKOUTS

Did you know that 60 per cent of your body's muscle mass is in your butt and thighs? So working these muscle groups regularly really gets your metabolism firing! This workout is designed make you sweat, targeting your butt, thighs, quads, hamstrings, calves and more, to help tone and work your lower body, HARD!

WORKOUT 1

Perform each exercise for 1 minute with a 10 second rest between exercises.
Complete the entire circuit 4 times.

1. MID SQUAT WITH FORWARD JAB

Keep your stance wide and deep with your toes pointing outwards. Engage your core and punch with power!

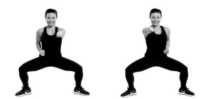

2. JUMPING SCISSOR LUNGE

Sink into a lunge, then use an explosive movement to jump and switch legs, sinking into a lunge on the other leg. Repeat. Make sure your knee doesn't extend past your front toe.

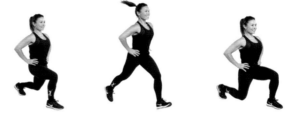

3. LUNGE PULSES

Take a big, long step forward, dropping the back knee close to the ground and pulse up and down. To avoid injury, make sure your front knee does not extend beyond your toe. Pump on one leg for one round and then alternate legs for the next round.

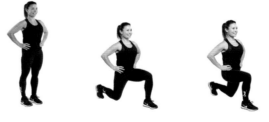

4. MOUNTAIN CLIMBER

Start in plank position and alternate bringing each knee in towards your chest. Focus on keeping your body in a straight line.

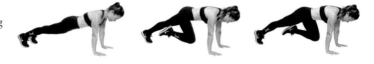

5. BRIDGE ON TOES

Lay on your back and squeeze those glutes as you lift your hips off the floor and come up onto your toes.

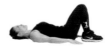

WORKOUT 2

**Perform each exercise for 1 minute with a 10 second rest between exercises.
Complete the entire circuit 4 times.**

1. ### SLOW JOG

Keep your head up and shoulders back as you jog on the spot.

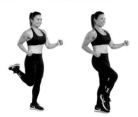

2. ### SIDE STEP UP

Focus on keeping the movement slow and controlled. Bring one foot onto the step and bring the other foot up to meet it. Step down and repeat. Alternate sides on each round.

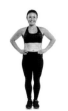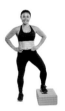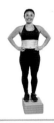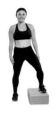

3. ### LUNGE PULSES

Take a big, long step forward, dropping the back knee close to the ground and pulse up and down. To avoid injury, make sure your front knee does not extend beyond your toe. Pump on one leg for one round and then alternate legs for the next round.

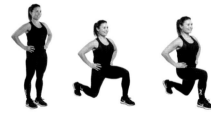

4. ### MOUNTAIN CLIMBER

Start in plank position and alternate bringing each knee in towards your chest. Focus on keeping your body in a straight line.

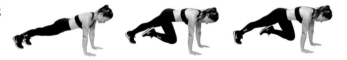

5. ### GLUTE SWING

Make sure your hips stay square and your back is in good alignment. Extend one leg out behind you. Swing your knee through towards your nose then push your foot back toward the roof. Repeat on the other side.

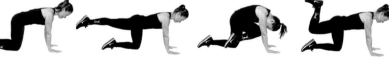

LOW IMPACT 20 MINUTE BUTT AND THIGH WORKOUT

The low impact variation of the butt and thigh workout is suitable for women recovering from a C-section or those with abdominal separation and/or a weak pelvic floor.

LOW IMPACT VARIATION

Perform each exercise for 1 minute with a 10 second rest between exercises. Complete the entire circuit 4 times.

1. PELVIC TILT WITH ARM RAISE

Contract your pelvic floor muscles and imagine moving your pubic bone towards your belly button. Lift your arms as you tilt your pelvis.

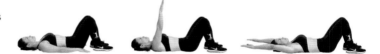

2. GLUTE SWING

Make sure your hips stay square and your back is in good alignment. Extend one leg out behind you. Swing your knee through towards your nose then push your foot back toward the roof. Repeat on the other side.

3. WINDSHIELD WIPER

Start in table-top position. Using a controlled movement, lower both legs to one side. Return them to the centre and repeat on the other side. Keep your core engaged.

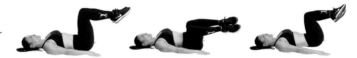

4. TOE TAPS

Start on your back with your legs in table-top position. Engage your core and tap your toes on the floor using slow, controlled movements, alternating left and right.

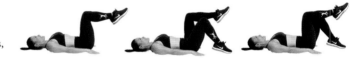

5. BICYCLE

Keep your core stable as you cycle your legs. Do this by drawing your navel in towards your spine.

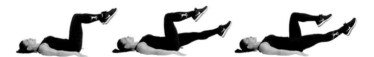

20 MINUTE FAT BLASTER WORKOUTS

We have created these 20 minute fat blaster workouts because we know that sometimes busy mums only have a little time to spare. A quick workout can still pack a metabolic punch – keep the intensity high when performing these workouts to get maximum bang for your 20-minute buck!

WORKOUT 1

**Perform each exercise for 1 minute with a 10 second rest between exercises.
Complete the entire circuit 4 times.**

1. PENDULUM

Focus on keeping your core engaged and your body upright as you swing your arms and one leg from side to side.

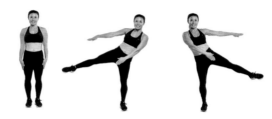

2. PUSH UP

Keep your body straight from toes to shoulders. Inhale and lower your body about 7–8 cm from the floor, keeping your elbows close to your body. Exhale, and push through the palms of your hands, returning to starting position.

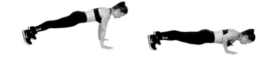

3. DANCING JACKS

Jump your legs out and raise your arms out in front, then jump back in. Jump your legs out again, but this time raise your arms out to the sides. Repeat.

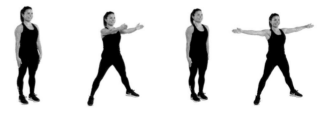

4. OVERHEAD JACKS

Keep your torso in alignment as you jump your legs out and raise your arms out to the side.

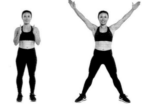

5. TRICEP DIP ON STEP

Keep your elbows in close to your body and lower your hips to the floor before pushing back up. Increase the challenge by moving your feet further out from the step.

WORKOUT 2

**Perform each exercise for 1 minute with a 10 second rest between exercises.
Complete the entire circuit 4 times.**

1. **OVERHEAD BALL THROW**

Keep your knees soft and bouncy, and take a shallow squat between each throw.

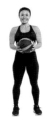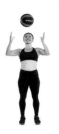

2. **SCISSOR JUMPS**

Jump your legs out with one in front of the other and, while swinging your arms, jump again to change feet. Repeat.

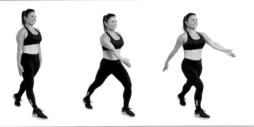

3. **BENT KNEE PUSH UP**

Keeping your back straight, bend your elbows until your chest is about 7–8 cm from the floor. Pause and push back to starting position.

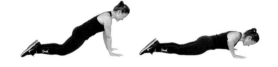

4. **SQUAT PUMPS**

Keep your attention on your core as you sink down into a squat position. Ensure your knees don't go past your toes and keep your back straight and shoulders back. Lift your arms in front of you and hold the squat position for 1–2 seconds, then gently pump up and down before returning to start position.

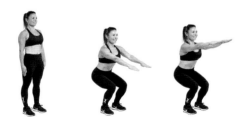

5. **BURPEE WITH LEG LIFT**

Place your hands on the floor in front of you, jump your feet out to plank position, then jump them back in and return to standing. Take a big jump, lifting your arms above your head, then lift one leg out to the side. Repeat the exercise on the other side.

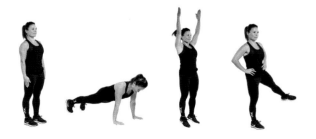

ACTIVE RECOVERY
DAY 1

It's important to include an active recovery day in your weekly exercise schedule, to allow time for your muscles to recover and repair, which helps to build strength. The stronger your muscles are, the more efficient your daily exercises will become.

We've suggested some light exercise options for the Active Recovery Days but you can choose anything you enjoy, such as walking, a gentle jog, playing with the kids at the park, yoga etc.

We've also included a suggested cardio and weight-based exercise for each recovery day, to keep you in the routine of being active. You can, of course, choose your own favourite cardio or weight-based exercise to perform as an alternative.

DAY 1

Light- to medium-intensity walk for 20 minutes or swim in the pool for 15 minutes followed by 10 minutes of light stretching.

PLUS: Low impact jacks for 2 minutes. Keep your torso in alignment and raise your arms out to the sides, as you step your legs out. Lower into a squat, then return to standing.

LOW IMPACT JACKS

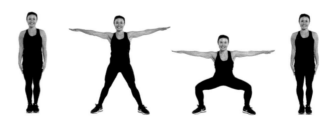

ACTIVE RECOVERY
DAY 2

DAY 2

Medium-intensity swim for 15 minutes or spend 20 minutes outdoors, throwing a ball or taking the dog for a walk.

PLUS: Alternating dumbbell shoulder press for 2 minutes. Hold a dumbbell in each hand with your elbows level with your shoulders. Alternate pushing the dumbbells into the air.

ALTERNATING DUMBBELL SHOULDER PRESS

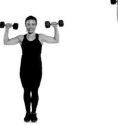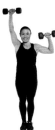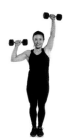

COOL DOWN

A cool down with gentle stretches will help minimise muscle soreness and tightness following your workout. Warm ups and cool downs are extra important following birth as your muscles and ligaments are strengthening and moving back into place.

You can either complete all of the cool-down exercises or choose 4–5 of them and perform for 4–5 minutes at the end of every workout. Hold each stretch for about 30 seconds.

1. SHOULDER STRETCH

Pull one arm across your body and use the opposite hand to apply pressure to your elbow, until you feel a stretch in your shoulder. Repeat on the other side.

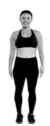 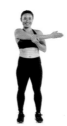 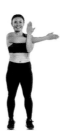

2. CHEST STRETCH

Stand tall and take your arms out to the sides at shoulder height, with palms facing up. You should feel a lovely stretch across the front of your chest.

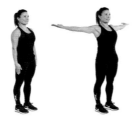

3. TRICEP STRETCH

Apply pressure to the elbow and reach your hand down between your shoulder blades, until you feel a gentle stretch along your tricep. Repeat on the other side.

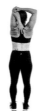 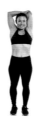

4. LYING QUADRICEP STRETCH

Focus on pressing your hips forward and keeping your knees in alignment. Pull one leg back and hold your ankle to feel the stretch in your quadricep. Repeat on the other side.

 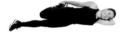

5. LYING HAMSTRING STRETCH

Bring your leg up as far as you can while keeping your knee straight. Only pull the leg towards you enough to feel a gentle stretch. Repeat on the other side.

 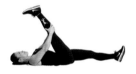

6. LYING GLUTE STRETCH

Place one foot on the other knee and hold your hands under the knee of the bottom leg. Pull gently and lift your foot off the ground.

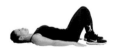 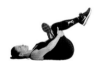

7. BABY POSE

Sink right back onto your feet and stretch your arms forward. Focus on relaxing completely.

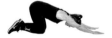 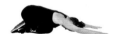

THANK YOU

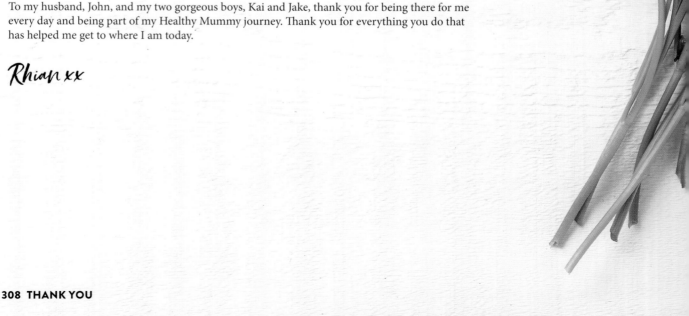

Without the help of the following fabulous people, none of this would have been possible:

The amazing team at Plum and Pan Macmillan, especially Lucy Heaver and Mary Small, your guidance and expertise to bring this book to life is truly appreciated.

The wonderful creative team: photographer Steve Brown, chef Sarah Mayoh, food stylist Vanessa Austin and designer Kirby Armstrong – wow! What an incredible job you've done to develop my ideas into beautiful pictures and designs.

My team of nutritionists, including Cheree Sheldon, Elisha Danine, Nikki Boswell and Sarina Darenzo – thank you for your guidance and skill in coming up with some of the yummiest and easiest-to-prepare healthy meals for all our busy mums!

Wendy Smith and Marissa Nieves, thank you for your fitness expertise, advice and suggestions. I love being able to work with some of the best in their field.

Marlene from Gasbag PR, thank you for shouting The Healthy Mummy message from the rooftops!

To my Healthy Mummy team of staff who dedicate so much of their time to share and grow this incredible business – thank you for your enthusiasm, love and support. A special thank you to Georga Holdich and Rachael Javes for being a huge part of creating this awesome book.

Thank you to The Healthy Mummy community of hundreds of thousands of busy mums; what can I say other than you guys are the best! Without you, The Healthy Mummy wouldn't exist and your passion for the business and support for each other never goes unnoticed.

To my husband, John, and my two gorgeous boys, Kai and Jake, thank you for being there for me every day and being part of my Healthy Mummy journey. Thank you for everything you do that has helped me get to where I am today.

Rhian xx

INDEX

A PLUM BOOK

First published in 2018 by Pan Macmillan Australia Pty Limited
Level 25, 1 Market Street, Sydney, NSW 2000, Australia
Level 3, 112 Wellington Parade, East Melbourne, Victoria 3002, Australia

Design by Kirby Armstrong
Photography by Steve Brown and Rob Palmer
Prop and food styling by Vanessa Austin
Edited by Rachel Carter
Index by Frances Paterson
Colour reproduction by Splitting Image Colour Studio
Printed and bound in China by 1010 Printing International Limited

A CIP catalogue record for this book is available from the National Library of Australia.

We advise that the information contained in this book does not negate personal responsibility on the part of the reader for their own health and safety. It is recommended that individually tailored advice is sought from your healthcare or medical professional. The publishers and their respective employees, agents and authors are not liable for injuries or damage occasioned to any person as a result of reading or following the information contained in this book.

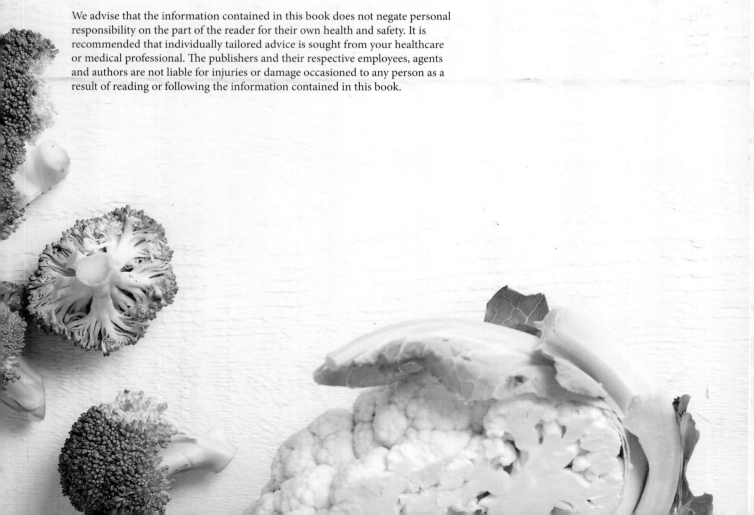